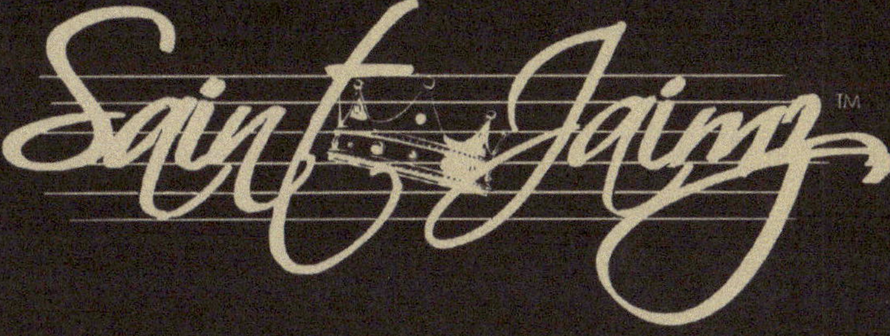

REVIVING THE ICONIC SOUND OF 90'S R&B

"THROWBACK, THE COVERS" VOL.1 A COMPILATION OF THE MOST TIMELESS 90'S R&B TRACKS

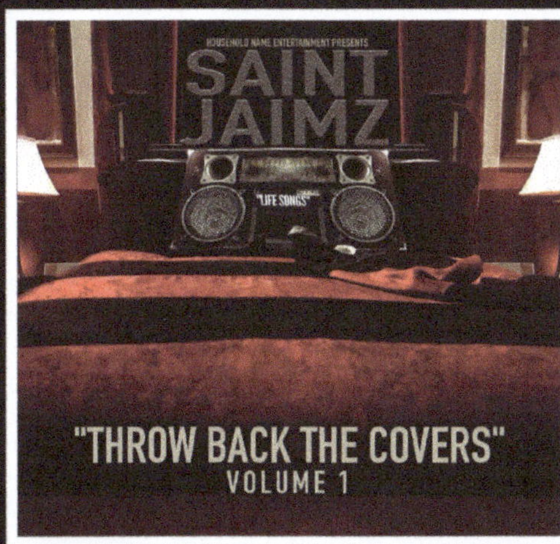

www.SaintJaimz.com

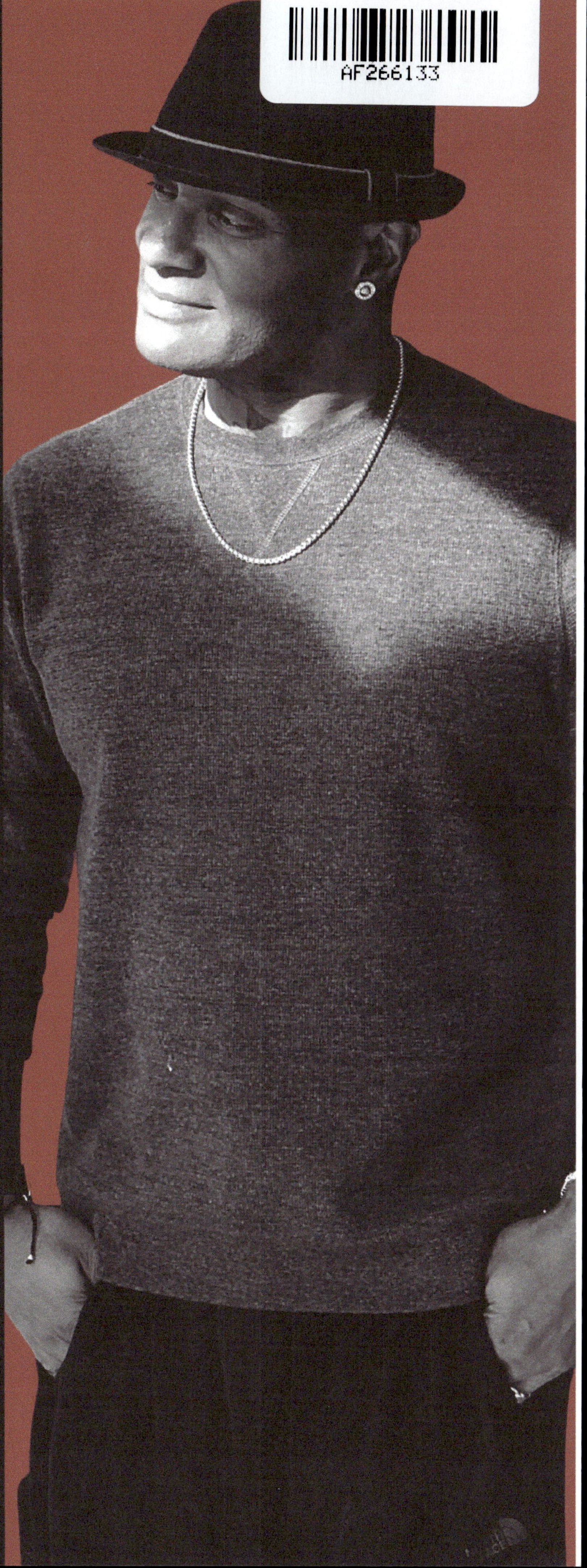

Pump it up Magazine

TABLE OF CONTENTS

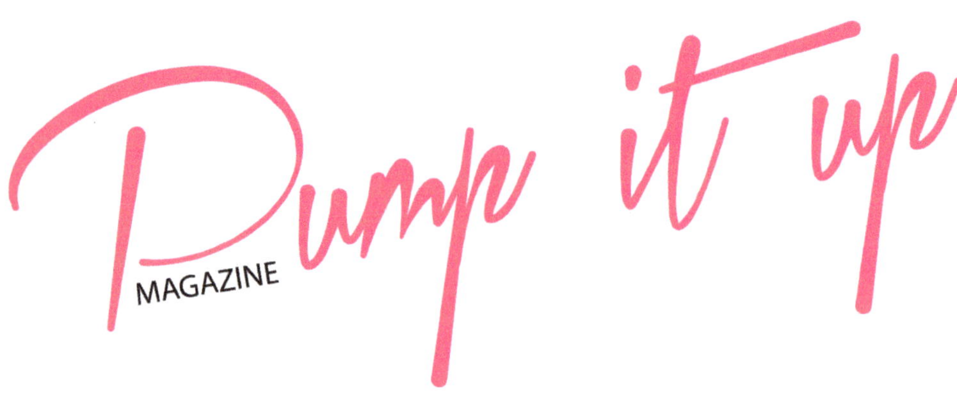

PUMP IT UP MAGAZINE

LINKS

WEBSITE
www.pumpitupmagazine.com

FACEBOOK
www.facebook.com/pumpitupmagazine

TWITTER
www.twitter.com/pumpitupmag

SOUNDCLOUD
www.soundcloud.com/pumpitupmagazine

INSTAGRAM
pumpitupmagazine

PINTEREST
www.pinterest.com/pumpitupmagazine

PUMP IT UP MAGAZINE
30721 Russell Ranch Road
Suite 140
Westlake Village,
California 91362
United States
www.pumpitupmagazine.com
info@pumpitupmagazine.com
Tel : (001) (877)841 – 7414 (toll free number)

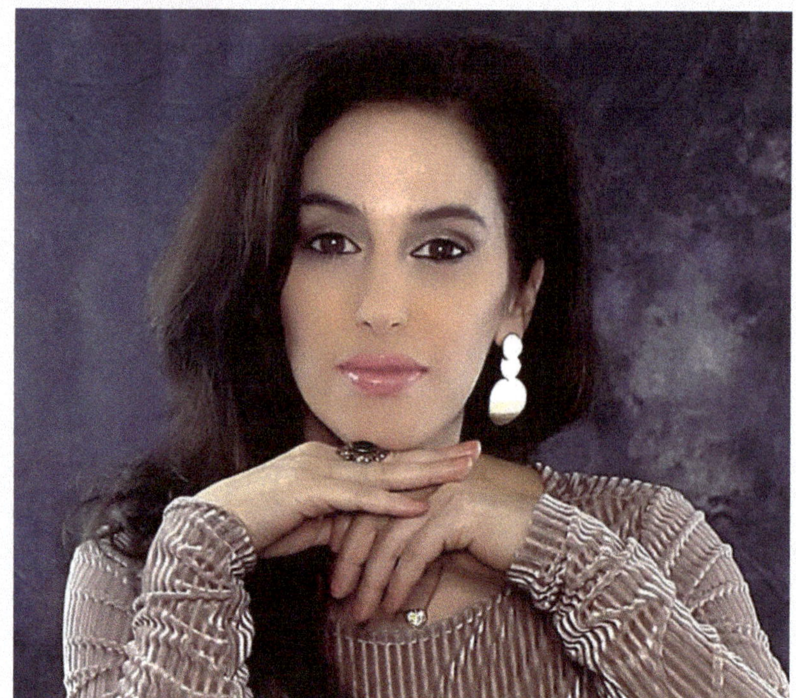

Greetings Readers,

Is Spring really here? Wow! how time flies when we are partially locked down in this Covid era. But there is light at the end of the tunnel so hang in there and observe the logic of events unfold hopefully in a positive way for all.

On the cover, rising R&B icon Saint Jaimz launches back onto the global music scene with his latest unforgettable EP "Throw Back the Covers (Vol. 1). The six-track epic is a compilation of the most timeless R&B tracks to grace us over the past few decades. "Throwback, The Covers" (Vol.1) is moving up the charts.

We have new music by amazing indie artists, and EM (our November 2020 cover girl) 's single Say What You Mean is now on Billboard charts among mainstream royalties!

Last but not least, I am happy to announce the release of my first Smooth Jazz album in America. It's called "Satisfied" I hope you will like it. You may pre-order CD and or Vinyl on my website www.Aneessa.com

Musicians and Artists, be sure to read about NFT's. It's overtaking the Music Industry

As usual, we have our Beauty section with Anti-aging secrets.

Our Fashion section is all about the '90s.

There are more Music industry tips and music documentaries to check out and in our humanitarian awareness section we bring your attention to the sensitive and caring subject of Autism with a focus on World Autism Awareness Day, April 2, 2021

So, flip through the pages of this edition and, don't forget to tune in to Pump It Up Magazine Radio where all the hits are played, and listen to our independent Spotify Playlist who has gathered more than 13k followers!

Be safe and be blessed!!

Anissa Boudjaoui

CONTRIBUTORS

EDITOR IN CHIEF
Anissa Boudjaoui

MUSIC
Michael B. Sutton
A. Scott Galloway
Sarah Kaye

FASHION
Tiffani Sutton

MARKETING
Grace Rose

PARTNERS

Editions L.A.
www.editions-la.com

The Sound Of L.A.
www.thesoundofla.com

Info Music
www.infomusic.fr

Delit Face
www.DelitFace.com

L.A. Unlimited
www.launlimitedinc.com

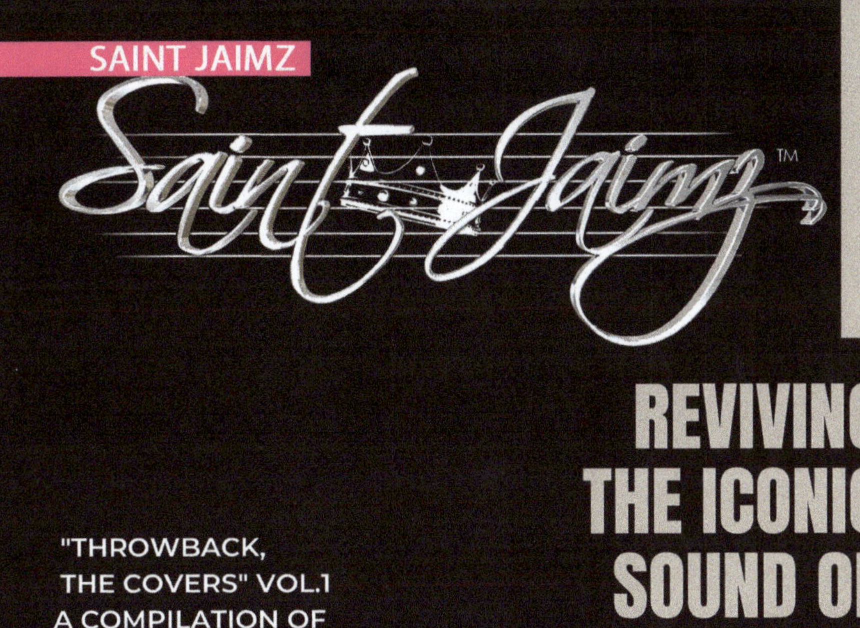

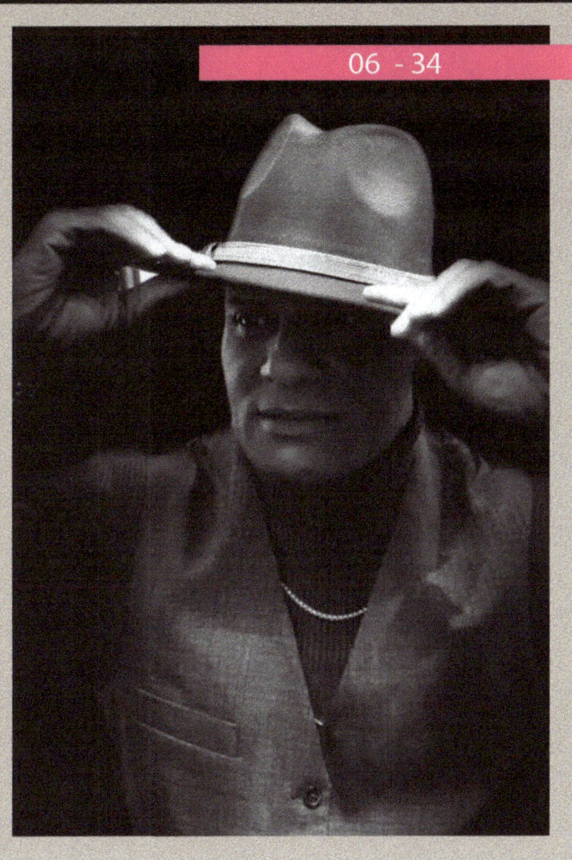

REVIVING THE ICONIC SOUND OF 90'S R&B

"THROWBACK, THE COVERS" VOL.1 A COMPILATION OF THE MOST TIMELESS 90'S R&B TRACKS

Based in California, singer – songwriter – producer Saint Jaimz has overcome incredible obstacles in order to follow his musical journey. A 16 year U.S Army Veteran, Jaimz served his country with great pride. *"The army is where I got my start in recording & singing live." says Saint Jaimz.* It is because of a military talent show in Germany, that he is involved in the music business today. Once you initially listen to Saint Jaimz's vocals, you are immediately taken aback to the legendary R&B slow jams of the 90's. He is amazing! His creative approach to marketing have allowed him to entertain many offers from the biggest moguls in the business. Once you've heard him, you are hooked!

Rapidly rising R&B icon Saint Jaimz launches back onto the global music scene with his latest unforgettable EP "Throw Back the Covers (Vol. 1). The six-track epic is a compilation of the most timeless R&B tracks to grace us over the past few decades. He really does justice to the classic sound of this brilliant genre by putting his own fresh spin on every song. It's brimming with positive energy and a softly soothing sound that really draws you straight into his world. The way he sings is so intimate it feels like we're right there with him. The kind of versatile vocals that soothe the soul and send us to a nicer place.

Opening up with the classic "Being Gentle", he really opens up strongly. With a gorgeous duet with up and comer "Sene" that really pulls on the heartstrings. It's the perfect bittersweet anthem for anyone that's gone through the rollercoaster of love. Next we are brought into luscious emotion-drenched soundscapes in "Baby Come Back". It's a cry out to that special someone in his life that he can't live without. The potently perfect song for anyone missing that person they cherish the most. It has a distinct catchy pop feel to it that makes it memorable. "Rock Wi'tcha" is more electronic-fuelled as we are taken on a journey through complex rhythms and smooth soundscapes.

Sene comes back in "Baby Come To me", an unforgettable duet that really sweeps you off your feet. The fierce female singer really takes centre stage in this one as she soothes us with mesmerizing melodies. Up and coming icon Kaleo Ross makes an appearance in the next track "Who Do You Love". It perfectly blurs the line between the more modern beat-driven style and the heartfelt bars of classic R&B. Truly a track that would be accessible to fans young and old. We finish up on "If You Were Here Tonight", a luscious layered harmonic track that tells a deep story. It's the kind of song that if you really focus on the lyrics you can feel the artist's pain. Overall it's a boundary breaking release that would appeal to R&B fans of all eras. Whether you're looking for that fix of the classic sound or looking for something more fresh, there's something to enjoy in this beautiful record.

Saint Jaimz is a Lover of Music and "Good" People.
His passion for music is his motivation and the inspiration behind his mission to bring R&B music back to the mainstream as a singer, songwriter, producer and CEO.

Since embarking upon the path of music, Saint Jaimz have made some remarkable accomplishments including Indie Soul Music Awards!

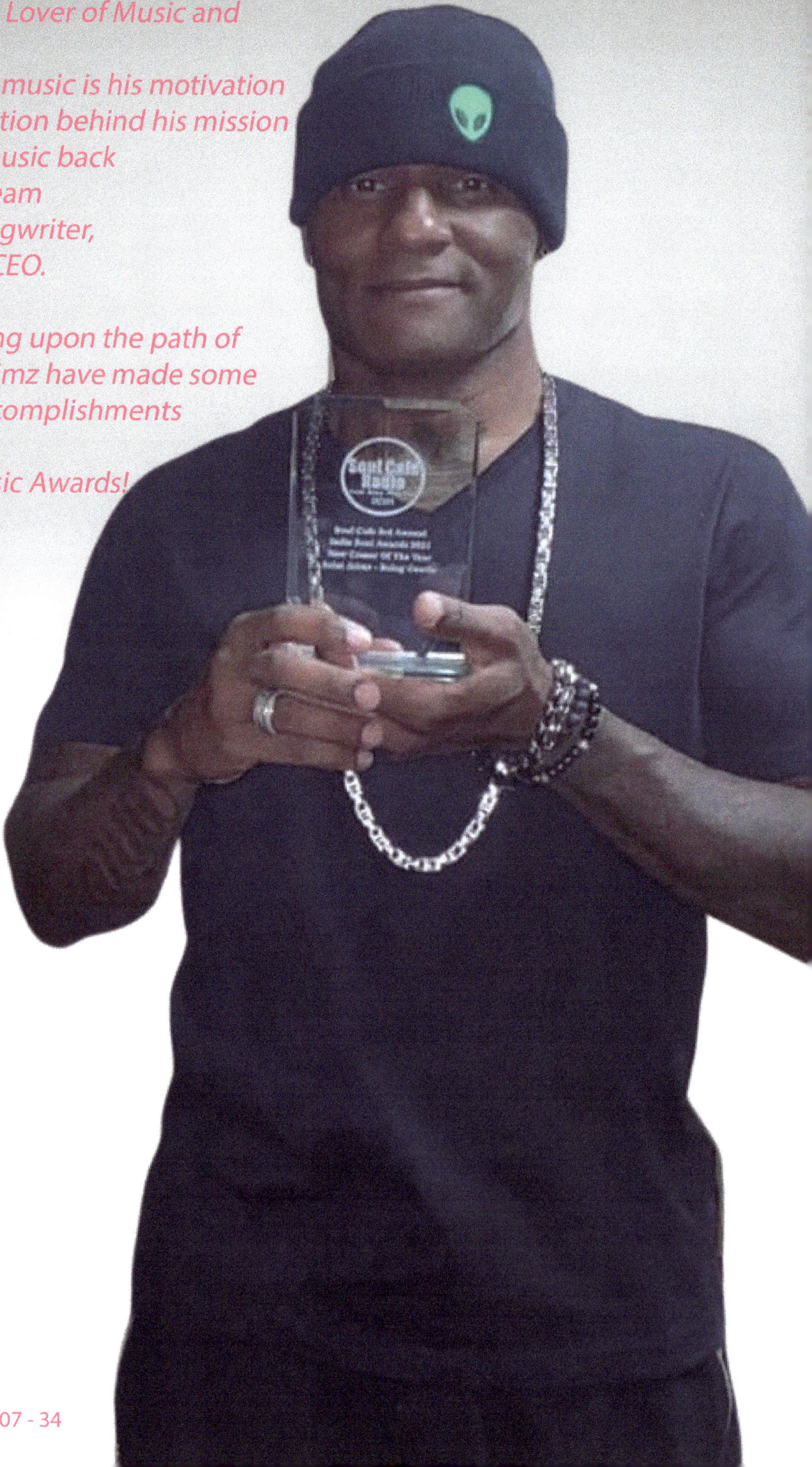

INTERVIEW WITH SAINT JAIMZ
R&B SINGER-SONGWRITER, PRODUCER
AND ENTREPRENEUR

As an entrepreneur, singer,songwriter, producer Saint Jaimz is a phenomenal individual and inspiring figure in the music world. His recent efforts have resulted in a fabulous EP titled Throw Back The Covers. In a recent conversation with Saint Jaimz, I got a chance to gain some insight into his background, musical experience, and the source of inspiration for his new project. I am sure you will find this interview enjoyable.

BEFORE WE BEGIN, I WOULD LIKE TO THANK YOU FOR TAKING THE TIME TO ANSWER A FEW QUESTIONS AND SHARE A GLIMPSE OF YOUR WORLD WITH OUR READERS. PLEASE INTRODUCE YOURSELF. WHO IS SAINT JAIMZ?

Saint Jaimz is a Lover of Music and "Good" People. His passion for music is his motivation and the inspiration behind his mission to Bring R&B music back to the mainstream as a singer, songwriter, producer and CEO. When He isn't making music, you will find him relaxing in his hot tub or working on new material and gearing up for the studio, or in a meeting connecting people and making moves that ultimately benefit the independent Artist.

WHAT WERE YOUR FORMATIVE YEARS LIKE AND HOW DID IT SHAPE YOUR PRESENT OUTLOOK ON THE WORLD?

My formative years were tough, I grew up in the City of Chicago where the average Black Person could barely afford to eat from month to month, so that taught you how to fight and be resilient ...Survival! I never want to go back to a place where I'm experiencing the inability to feed myself, my family, or to survive so, those formative years and being in those tough situations put me in a situation to be able to have the drive and the work ethic I have now. I always try to do what's best and do good Business.

WHAT INSPIRED YOU TO PURSUE THE PATH OF MUSIC

Growing up with a singing Grandmother. She was a Gospel Singer and of course she loved the classics. She would sing church music on Sunday and the Classics during the week, James Brown, Otis Redding, Sam Cook, The Temptations, and etc. I got my inspiration from my grandmother and which inspired me to love singing, the desire to create music and Art. As I got older wanting to be a part of the music industry, was always intriguing because of all the people that paved the way prior to me. Growing up watching these people do what they loved and be good at it, I wanted to be just like a lot of them, From Michael Jackson to Bruno Mars!

WHAT WERE SOME OF THE OBSTACLES THAT YOU HAD TO OVERCOME AND LESSONS LEARNED TO BECOME THE MAN YOU ARE TODAY?

Again, coming from poverty to stability I attribute the military for that. I went to the military right out of high school. The military helped me get on my feet and stabilize my mindset in life. The discipline I have now comes from that. Some obstacles have been from poverty, some from dealing with self-worth. I'm very transparent about my life, when you are young, black, and poor, somebody is always telling you, you aren't going to amount to much. Especially being black in America, you start believing that lie and end up not even trying or attempting to do any better.

I never felt like I was worthless, I just knew I didn't want to continue to go through the things I did while growing up, I wanted to have a better life for myself and when I had children, I wanted to provide a better life for them. So, the challenges were rough! Poverty, Education and just the challenge of being racially discriminated against was unimaginable.

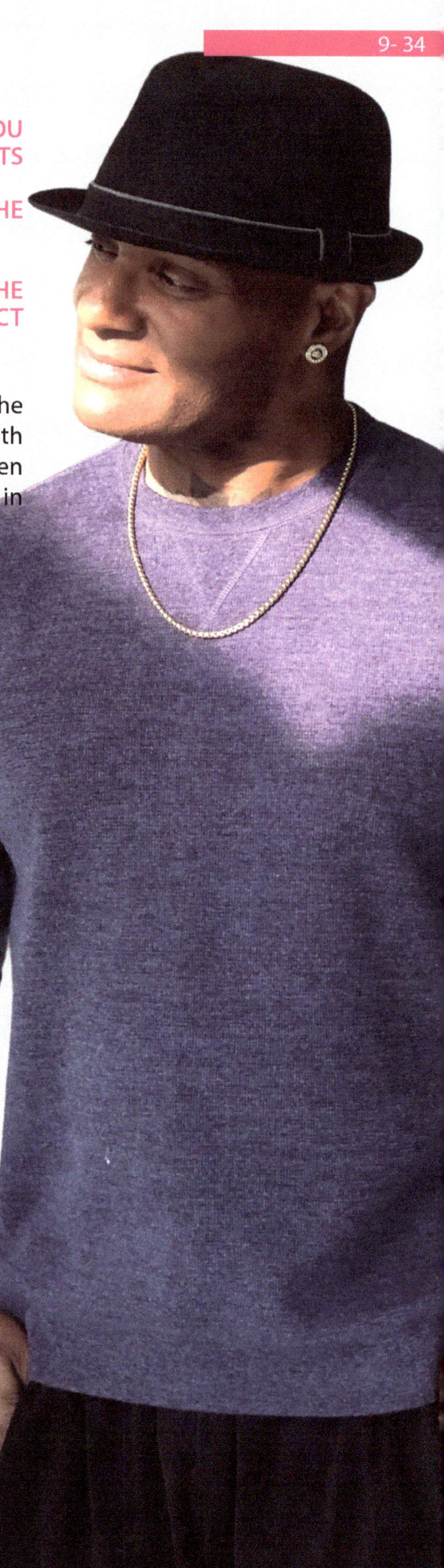

SINCE EMBARKING UPON THE PATH OF MUSIC, YOU HAVE MADE SOME REMARKABLE ACCOMPLISHMENTS INCLUDINGINDIE SOUL MUSIC AWARDS, AND THE RECENT RELEASE OF THE THROWNBACK THE COVERS (VOLUME 1).

CAN YOU TELL US A LITTLE BIT ABOUT THE AWARD, THE EP AND WHAT INSPIRED YOU TO RELEASE THE PROJECT AT THIS TIME?

The award was unexpected but definitely appreciated! The initiation into the indie world, these last 8 months, with people in the music world discovering what I've been knowing all along and doing all along, the music I have in my catalog being able to have people gravitate to it and appreciate it along with helping people through some tough times in their life with the type of songs I create, which are Life Songs. My peers voted for me to get that award, which to me helped solidify that okay, I'm starting to get attention from my peers.

The Throw Back The Covers EP is inspired because through this pandemic, you should not be doing the same thing you were doing pre-pandemic continue to do post-pandemic.

It's a whole different planet, whole different world, and country here in America. I felt like a throw back, nostalgic project taking people back to a place that rekindled some memories or reignited some passions with the type of songs I chose.

The songs I chose, I felt was really going to resonate with people. I told a lot of people before I did it that it was probably going to be dope and they shrugged it off but, look at it now. I'm really excited about it, I say that with all humility never arrogance.

I'm focused on providing good music and getting back to Classic and Solid R&B.

WHAT THEME WOULD YOU LIKE LISTENERS OF THROW BACK THE COVERS TO EMBRACE FROM THIS ENTHRALLING COLLECTION OF MUSIC?

More about nostalgia and rekindling peoples love for classic R&B and wanting them to remember what it felt like to hear a record and have to repeat it over and over and each time u hear, learn and love something more about it than before. and it be the soundtrack to your life. This Genre of music is reemerging and people are rekindling their relationship with Rhythm and Blues.

YOU HAVE ALSO FORMED AN INDEPENDENT LABEL NAMED HOUSEHOLD NAME ENTERTAINMENT. CAN YOU TELL US A BIT ABOUT THE COMPANY'S ORIGINS AND SOME OF THE ARTISTFEATURED?

The name Household Name came about because of my previous manager and partner used to say I'm going to be a household name one day. When I got to a place where I wanted to graduate from being just a recording artist to doing production and label type of work, and ultimately CEO type of business, that's when I decided my company should be Household Name Entertainment. I actually have the name Trademarked and the name Saint Jaimz. My name has been changed legally to Saint Jaimz. I have other Independent Artists I produce and partner with under "SAINT JAIMZ PRESENTS": I am partnering with artists and we are putting together Ep's, Singles, and Projects and just putting them out to the independent market. We are hoping to maintain some success with these projects, we have to keep Working an Striving!

We want to knock the door down. With the current traction, I have as an independent artist, I'm basically trying to bring people along with me that have the ability to really change the world with their music.

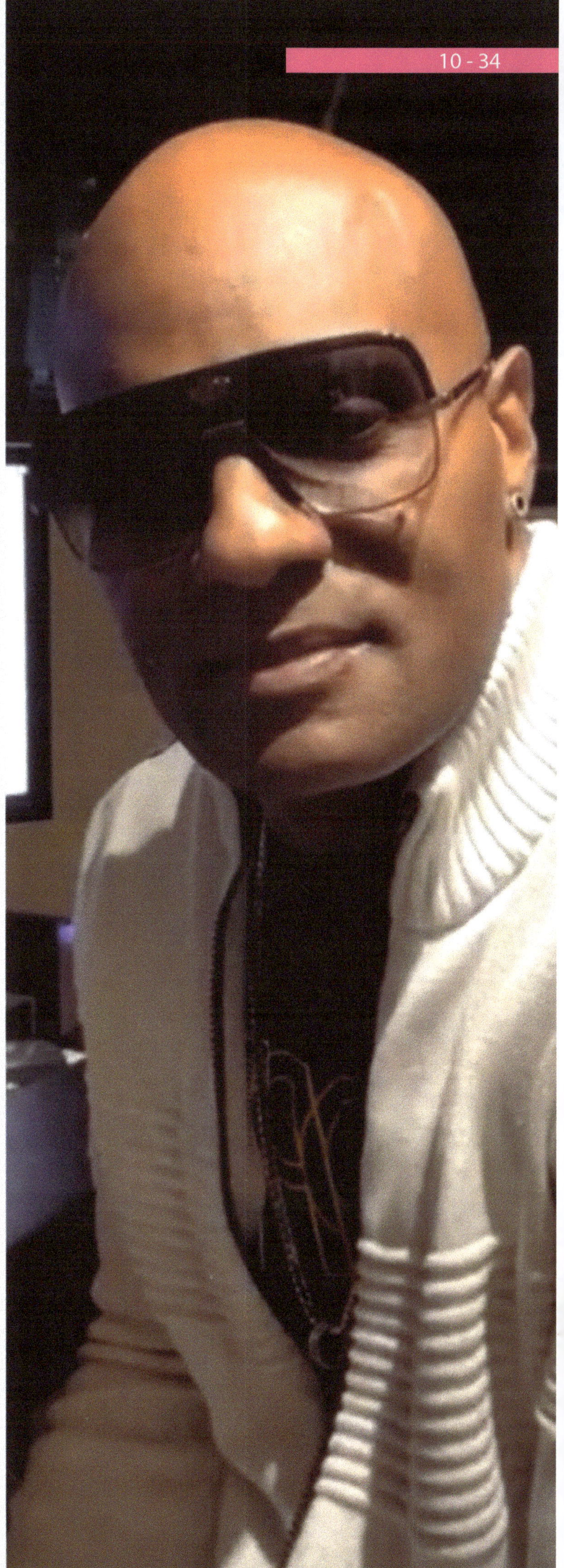

As an African American, I already understand the disparity among my people and the social-economic disadvantages in education, housing, healthcare and with food and dietary concerns. However, when it comes to Mental Health Issues and being born with Mental and Psychological Disabilities like Autism, race and all that other nonsensical politics goes out the window! Some Parents in my community have no idea what Autism is or that they need to have their child who may or may not be exhibiting signs of being Autisitc, evaluated and treatment. This has to be Addressed. As we already know, We are no longer treating our Mentally Challenged we are Incarcerating Them! So Please "GIVE" to Autism Speaks! Let's Change the World! One Kid at a time!

WHAT CAN WE EXPECT TO HEAR FROM SAINT JAIMZ IN THE NEAR FUTURE?
ANY FINAL THOUGHTS?

More and more R&B, that's my staple. I'm open to all genres and any artist that's willing to invest in themselves and want to work, do good business, and be treated with respect. Come talk to us at Household Name Ent. We want to partner with you and continue to put out great content and quality music. It has been a rough year for our Music Industry. A lot of us could barely afford to pay our bills let alone continue to create the music and content that so many people expect or desire without support. I would hope that people would begin to donate or give to organizations that help musicians, gig workers, and independent artists like myself, so that we can continue doing what we love, as doing what we love creates what you love and that's great music! I appreciate all the love and support out there and I'll continue to give it back\through my music. Thank you all so very much!

Thank you once again Saint Jaimz for taking the time out of your busy schedule to answer a few questions and share a glimpse of your life's work with our readers. I would like to wish you all the best in you artistic and personal endeavors.

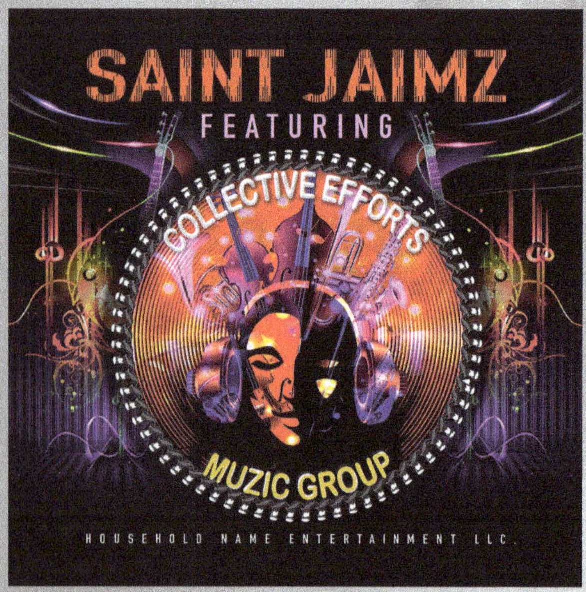

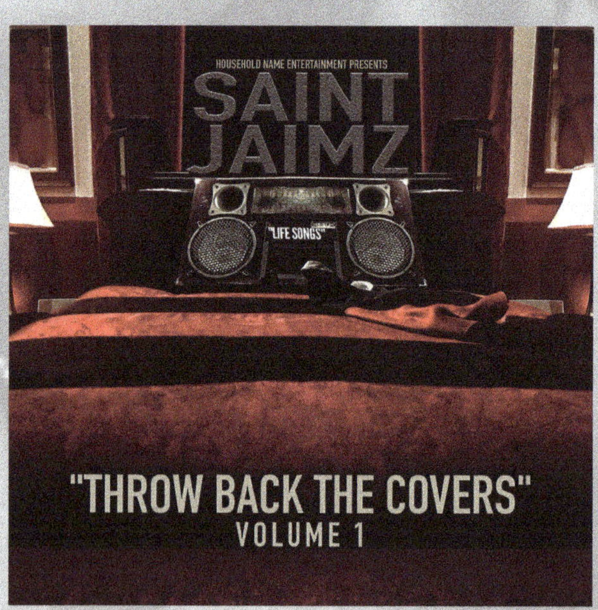

To know more about Saint Jaimz, please visit:

http://www.SaintJaimz.com

http://www.facebook.com/saintjaimz2

http://www.instagram.com/saintjaimz

http://www.twitter.com/saintjaimz916

Enjoy The Sound Of

Pump it up

RADIO

Get the free Pump it up magazine Radio App on your smartphone or tablet, and you'll never miss your favourite music !

POP - ROCK - DANCE - RNB - JAZZ
Available on Google Play Store

www.PumpItUpMagazine.com

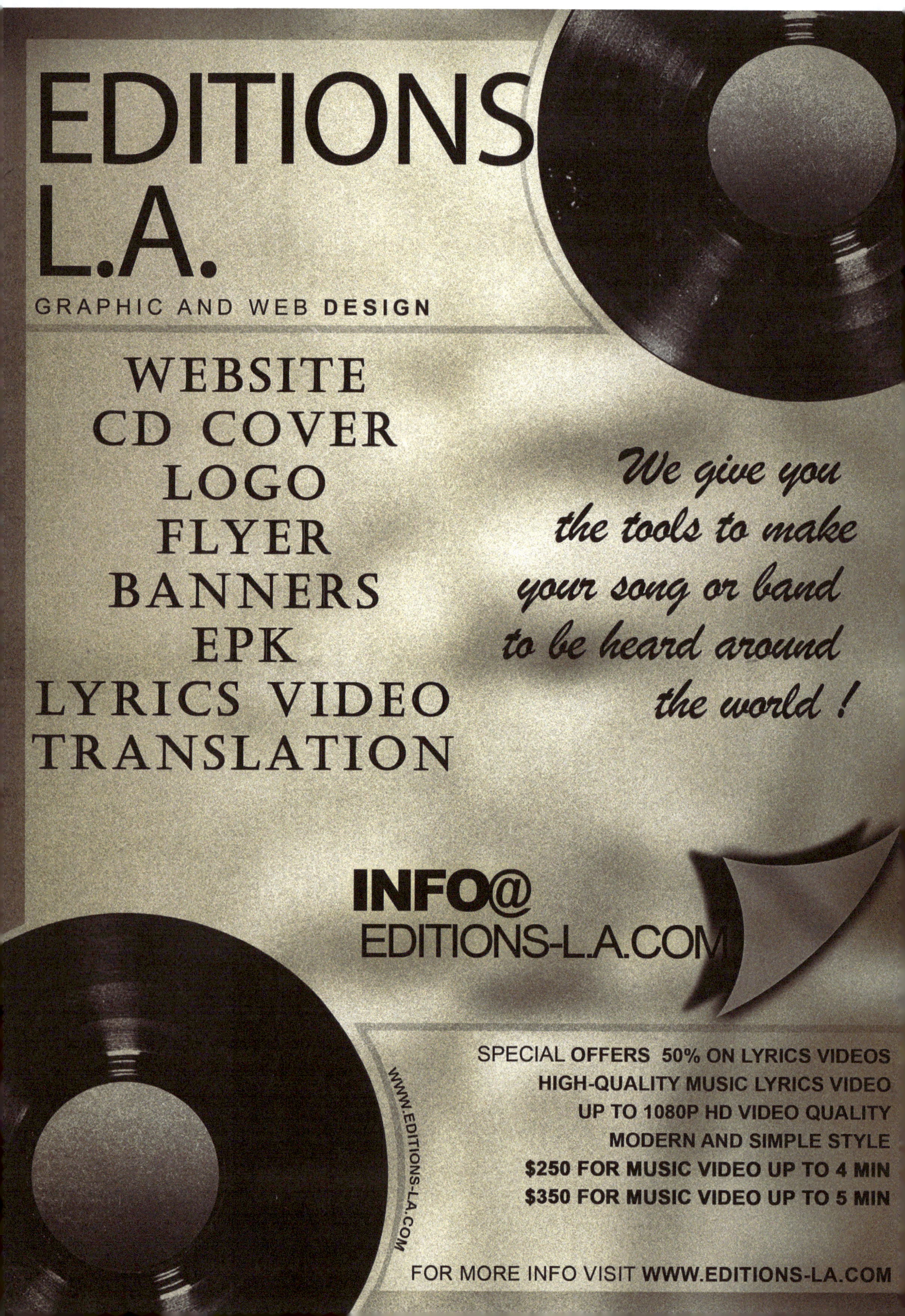

EDITIONS L.A.

GRAPHIC AND WEB **DESIGN**

WEBSITE
CD COVER
LOGO
FLYER
BANNERS
EPK
LYRICS VIDEO
TRANSLATION

We give you the tools to make your song or band to be heard around the world !

INFO@
EDITIONS-L.A.COM

WWW.EDITIONS-LA.COM

SPECIAL **OFFERS** 50% ON LYRICS VIDEOS
HIGH-QUALITY MUSIC LYRICS VIDEO
UP TO 1080P HD VIDEO QUALITY
MODERN AND SIMPLE STYLE
$250 FOR MUSIC VIDEO UP TO 4 MIN
$350 FOR MUSIC VIDEO UP TO 5 MIN

FOR MORE INFO VISIT WWW.EDITIONS-LA.COM

NFTS- NON-FUNGIBLE TOKENS OVERTAKING THE MUSIC INDUSTRY

Last week, rock band Kings of Leon became the first band to release an album as an NFT, expanding the possibilities for crypto and blockchain technology in the music industry. If that first sentence already lost you, you've come to the right place. NFTs are undoubtedly the buzziest new topic in music and for good reason. In February 2021 alone, NFTs earned nearly 22 million dollars in the music industry, according to data collected by Water & Music, but it's much like explaining the Internet to someone in the '90s who has never seen it before. NFTs are highly conceptual and unprecedented, but it makes sense once you get used to the idea.

Consider this article your true introductory guide to NFTs in the music business, wherein, we will break down the most important characteristics of the technology, its potential impacts on the industry (both positive and negative), and which musicians and companies are leading the space.

WHAT ARE NFTS?

A non-fungible token (NFT) is a form of cryptocurrency. Think of cryptocurrency as a fancy box that cannot be tampered with or broken into, and within that box, information can be securely placed inside. This box of information can hold just about anything: money, art, music, contracts, essays, etc. Many of us are already familiar with Bitcoin or Ethereum (or we have at least heard those terms float around for the last few years), and for those cryptocurrencies, money is placed safely inside the box. Money is considered "fungible," meaning its value is interchangeable with other monies. This means that exchanging Bitcoin is just like exchanging physical cash: a $20 bill can be traded for four $5 bills and a US dollar can be swapped for its equivalent in Mexican pesos. Bitcoin is easy to transfer with something that holds equal value.

Conversely, a non-fungible token (NFT), which we will focus on in this guide, is anything that is not easily interchangeable that is placed into that box. An equivalent to this in the real world is the Mona Lisa (or any other work of art). There is only one original copy of this painting, and it cannot be replicated no matter what happens. Someone could try to repaint the Mona Lisa or take a photo of it but that will never mean that it is the exact same as the original. Also, the non-fungible Mona Lisa will not lose value because someone has taken a photo of it or tried to paint it themselves. No one could ever replicate the artist's signature, the aging of the paint, the specific brush strokes made. All of these unique aspects make the Mona Lisa non-fungible by nature. Trading the Mona Lisa for another famous painting is difficult to reconcile because no painting is of exact equal value to another.

In the crypto space, an NFT can be art as well, but it can also be other unreplicable forms, including music, tickets, contracts, and more. That's where the music industry comes in, using this technology to create unique, sellable pieces of digital merchandise, art work, music and experiences to fans.

But first, what makes crypto so game-changing? Answer: its decentralization and its promise of security. Cryptocurrency was first invented in 2008 with the creation of Bitcoin, and it became revolutionary for cutting out the middleman in finance. In a typical cash system, societies rely on banks and governments to protect their monetary transactions, which can be costly and cumbersome to deal with. In situations like The Great Depression, this can even be dangerous when those institutions fail. Crypto is different because it uses blockchain technology — a publicly accessible ledger of all transactions with a certain "box." Each time a transaction occurs, a new block (or, per our analogy, a secure "box") is created, forming a chain of blocks over time that cannot be tampered with and that get more secure with each block added. These blocks store important information like time stamps of transactions and who and what has been exchanged. This is much more secure than our current system, which is fairly hackable in the digital age and relies on fallible middle men to control the ledger. In contrast, to hack a blockchain, one would have to alter every single block on the chain, one by one, making it far more impervious than traditional banking. Funny enough, this logic is a lot like a fancy form of "Car Fax", which acts as a transparent record of all prior use of a vehicle.

HOW ARE NFTS SOLD?

NFTs can be sold on crypto-marketplaces. Overwhelmingly, music NFTs are sold using an auction or silent auction model (think, a digital form of Sotheby's or Christie's), but some are sold at a set price instead. It is up to the seller which method is preferred. Most marketplaces do not accept credit cards or traditional forms of cash and instead ask for cryptocurrencies, but there are a few that accept both traditional cash and cryptocurrency.

WHO YOU SHOULD KNOW IN THE WORLD OF MUSIC NFTS

One of the best ways to understand music industry NFTs is to look at a few key early players in the space, pioneering music NFTs as their popularity rapidly expands. In fact, sales of music NFTs have reportedly grown 150 times over the last six months, according to data from Water & Music, and it seems that nowadays every artist (and music company) is trying to get in on the hype.

NFTs in the music industry can take on many forms, including but not limited to ticket sales for concerts (virtual and physical), sample packs, previews of unreleased songs, art, and more. With such growth, it can be anticipated that potential uses for this technology will expand quickly and reach far beyond how the industry utilizes NFTs today.

ARTISTS

For artists, NFTs offer the exciting possibility of cutting out some of the industry's middlemen and monetizing their work in brand-new ways. Mike Shinoda, co-founder of Linkin Park, for example, raised $30,000 auctioning a 37-second teaser of an unreleased song, paired with an animation of a skull as an audio-visual NFT. In a Twitter thread explaining the move, Shinoda noted, "Think of it like owning a 1 of a kind item in a game … It's a weird thing to own, yes, but: Here's the crazy thing. Even if I upload the full version of the contained song to DSPs worldwide (which I can still do), I would never get even close to $10k, after fees by DSPs, label, marketing, etc." For most established artists with sizable teams, like Shinoda, managers, labels, publishers, co-writers, and more take percentages of the artists' profits from their music, leaving artists with small fragments of the money their work has earned.

Though electronic artists are the most common early adopters, like top earners 3LAU and Deadmau5, musicians across genres are joining the trend, including the aforementioned rock group Kings of Leon, who dropped the first album ever as an NFT last week. Released via YellowHeart, an NFT marketplace that counts The Chainsmokers as partners, the group is not only offering the album itself as an NFT; it also offers digital artwork and six "golden tickets," all as NFTs. If a fan gets the golden ticket, they can redeem "four front-row tickets at any Kings of Leon headline show, anywhere in the world, once per tour." In this case, the NFT's blockchain technology allows for a secure transfer of the golden ticket directly into the fan's digital wallet. The album NFT itself will be available for purchase for two weeks, and it will include digital album artwork, one full digital album download, and a physical copy of a limited-edition vinyl.

This also opens up possibilities for producers. Grammy-nominated producer Illmind recently offered up the world's first sample beat pack as an NFT, announcing it via Twitter on February 25th. Anyone can listen to the beat pack, but ownership and the rights to use the pack only go to the highest bidder. This sale in particular could have a major impact on the way music is licensed and sold. Currently, licensing music or transferring ownership is an inconvenient process for labels, publishers and their lawyers, often resulting in pushed-back release dates as people work to manually clear each sample use or transfer of ownership. With NFTs, it is as quick as buying just about anything else online, and the technology allows for clear documentation of the transfer.

DELIT FACE

Social Media For The Entertainment World

MUSIC & MOVIE Industry

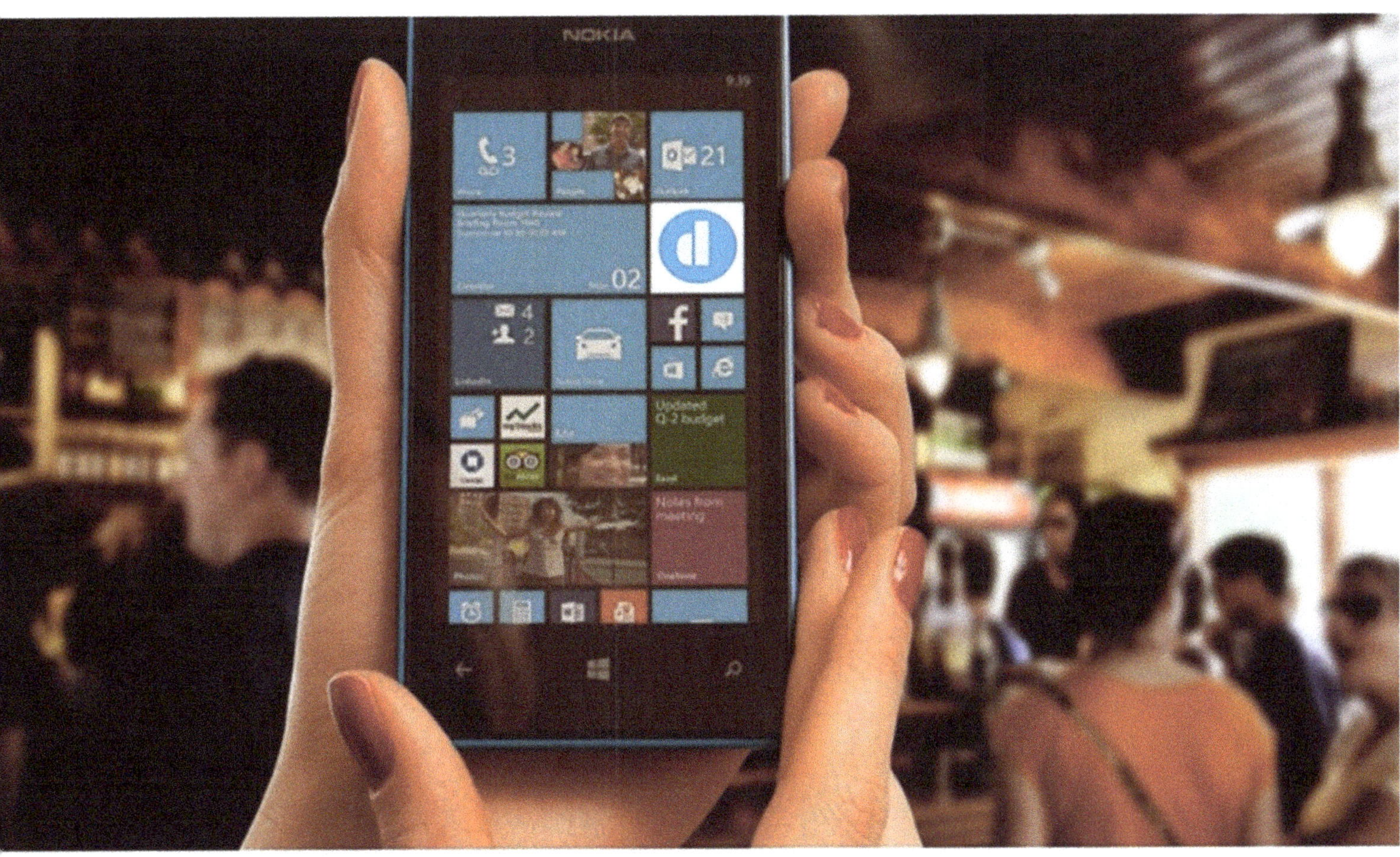

SINGER
SONGWRITER
MUSICIANS
PRODUCERS
PUBLISHERS
DISTRIBUTORS
MUSIC SUPERVISORS

ACTORS
DIRECTORS
PRODUCERS
DISTRIBUTORS
SET DESIGNERS
SCRIPT
WRITERS
EXTRAS

MAKE UP ARTISTS
HAIR STYLISTS
PHOTOGRAPHERS
GRAPHIC DESIGNER

Register now FREE and connect with people in your industry

www.delitface.com

MICHAEL "MICKY" SCHUMAN

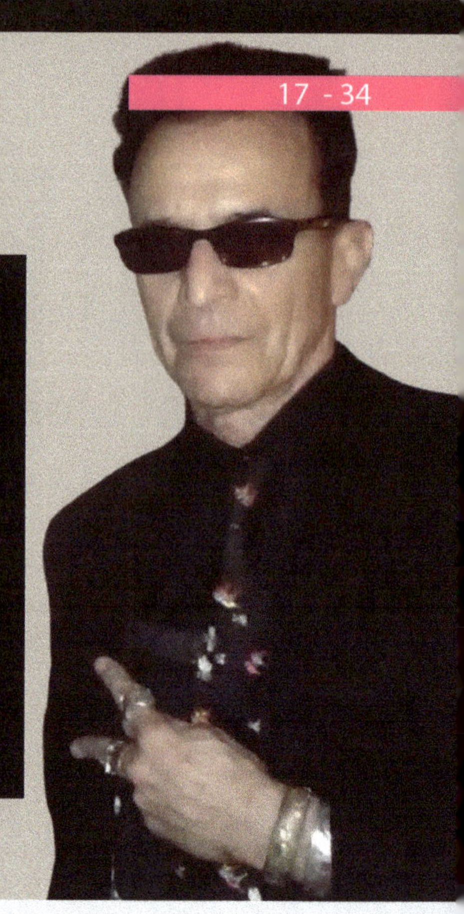

MUSICIAN
SONGWRITER
RECORDING ENGINEER
PRODUCER

THE JACK OF ALL TRADES

"I have been Lucky to work with so many talented artists and musicians and I am so Thankful. Great memories. Great friendships!"

We had held an exclusive interview with Michael Schuman few days ago where Michael told us about his beginning in the music industry, how he started learning drums from the master himself, Chuck Flores of Professional Drums, at 8 years old. At 11 years old, he was already a violinist, playing piano, writing music, and was performing at parties with his 16-year-old band-mates.

The veteran music producer was 12 when he got his first go at recording in an actual studio. Before that, he wanted to be a lawyer cum Olympic gymnast rather than a professional in the entertainment industry. His parents didn't share his enthusiasm and tried to discourage him during his high school years, doing their best to make him realize how hard it was to be a music professional. However, for Michael, the vibe that echoed in the recording studio was everything. He could live there.

"The recording studio itself; the smell of the wood, the cork on the walls, the sounds, the vibe that echoed.... I needed no encore. This is where I need to be. That was it. I didn't know what "it' was... but I knew it", said Michael.

When asked about being a recording engineer, this California based star replied that this transformation was as natural as the circle of life. His fascination with recording sounds eventually evolved into music. Michael's first job at Fidelity Recorders was where he cut his teeth and met successful artists like Alan Oday, Steven Bishop, Mike and Brenda Sutton, to name a few.

Working with Mike and Brenda Sutton on Smokey Robinson's albums is one of Mr. Schuman's fondest memories.

Artists build their dreams and create their world on the foundation of producing music; this producer added when enquired about his production projects. According to Michael, he realized that he built a platform where icons are made after being in awe of the music industry. It was his collaboration with other artists that launched his career as a producer. Michael believes that the evolution of music took a very different route from what he anticipated. Though he likes some of the new songs and thinks some artists do have that "IT" factor. While talking about new platforms and resources, the experienced producer added that the new platforms do fulfill the need of those whose souls yearn for music. The producers and DJs are thought of as the new artists of today.

"I have been Lucky to work with so many talented artists and musicians and I am so Thankful. Great memories. Great friendships", said Michael.

In response to our question on opting a professional studio over home-based set-up, the world leading artist said that a professional studio has the edge over a home recording set-up as artists can build chemistry all great bands have while playing simultaneously together, comfortably in a professional recording studio. For a producer and engineer, working with all the tools he needs in a real room is the Real Deal. Home-based set-up lacks that. It's good for recording a single instrument, but the vibe and result of people playing together is another dimension. He thinks he is spoiled by working in some of the greatest studios in the world.

Remembering his beginning, Mr. Schuman added nothing was digital at that time. Editing was done by a razor blade. They had to lock two machines together in order to get 48 tracks. The song he is working on nowadays has 200 stereo tracks. He said that learning within great limitations and no schooling gave him the best education with no boundaries. When asked about a good mix, Michael classified it as something that can move him regardless of him liking the lyrics or vocals. At the same time, a good master has it all, a Good Song (Lyric and Melody), a soulful vocal, then an excellent arrangement with fabulous production, mystical musical performances, perfect recording, mixing, and state-of-the-art mastering.

The visionary producer is currently working on a song he wrote about children and their empowerment, which involves a number of artists like Stevie Wonder and Paris Jackson. Another one of his songs is now featured in a Broadway musical about Elliot Willenky's life. Elliot wrote hit songs for Michael Jackson, Whitney Houston, Jermaine Jackson, etc. In addition to all above mentioned projects, *the star is also excited about the launch of a revolutionary mobile app which is being designed to give artists and everyone around the world a new platform to communicate, empower, and serving humanity.*

Contact this amazingly talented star, Michael "Micky" Schuman at MickyDelRey@gmail.com , 310 625 4681, or follow him at www.facebook.com/mickyschuman and https://www.linkedin.com/in/MichaelSchuman/

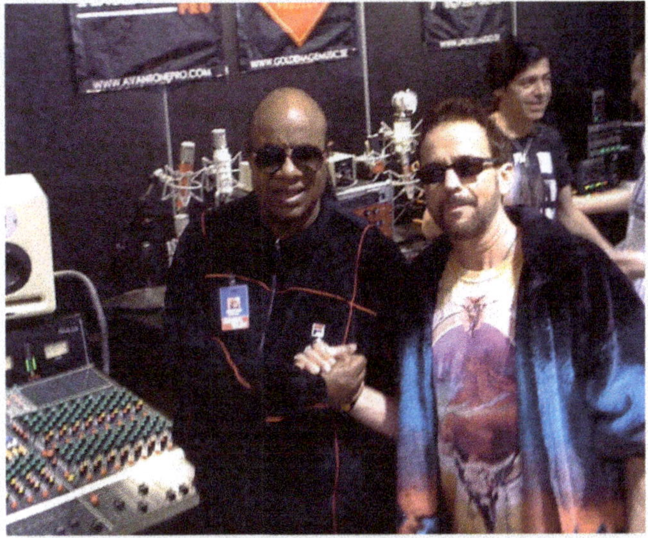
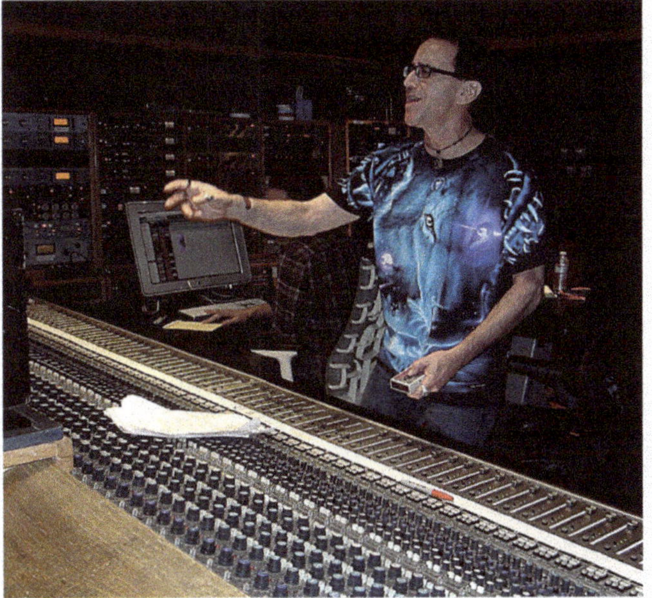
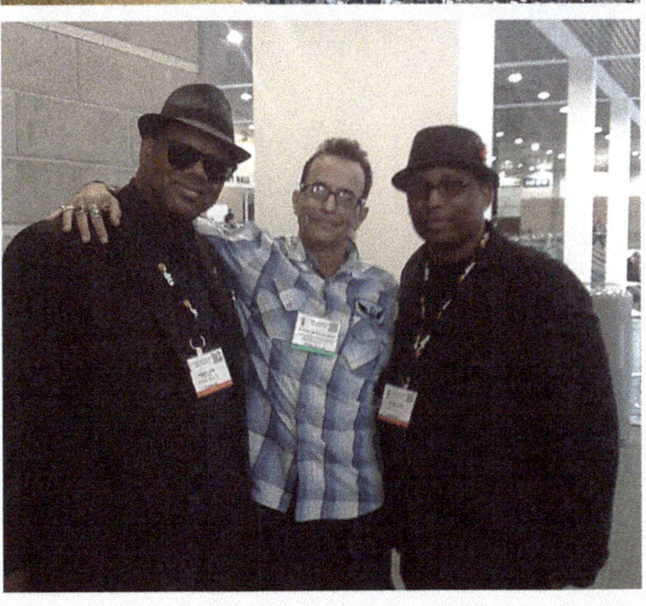

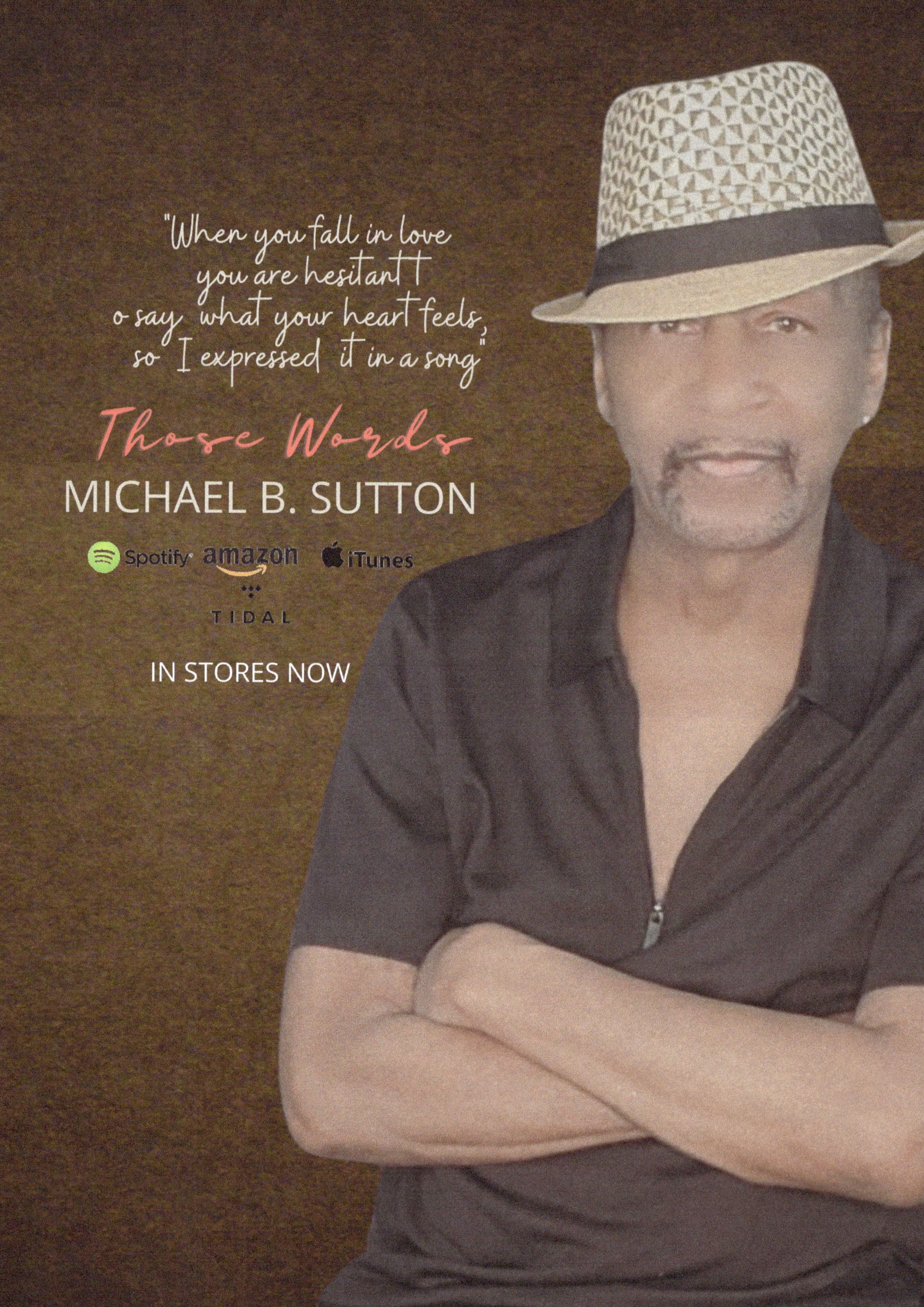

"When you fall in love
you are hesitant t
o say what your heart feels,
so I expressed it in a song"

Those Words

MICHAEL B. SUTTON

Spotify amazon   iTunes

TIDAL

IN STORES NOW

NICOLETTE SULLIVAN

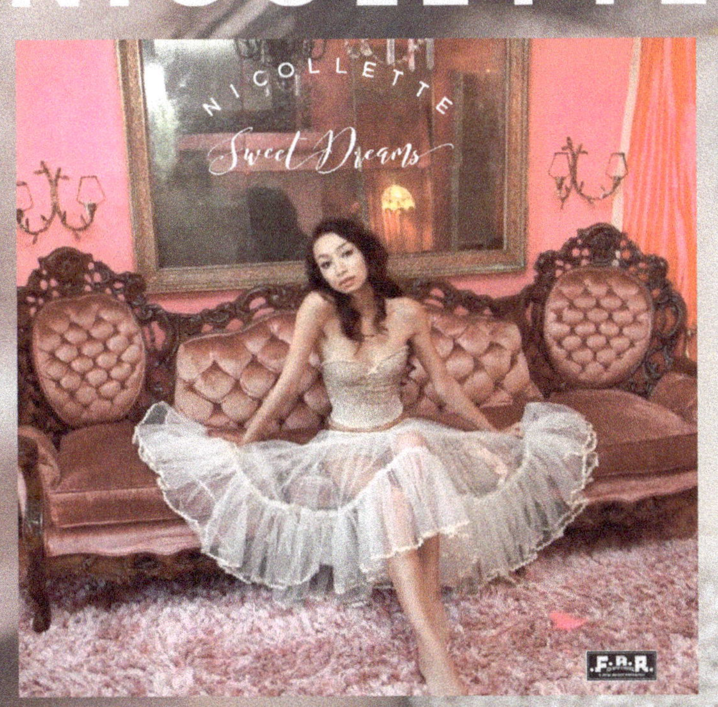

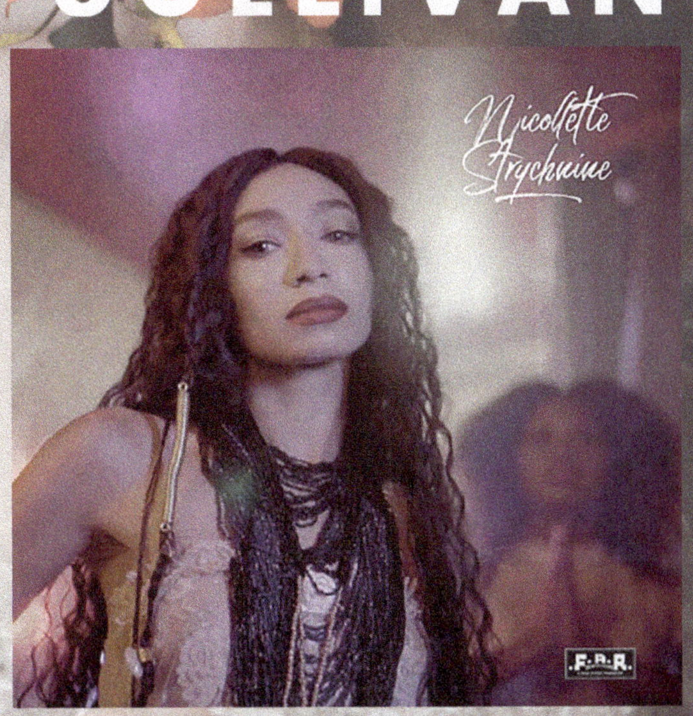

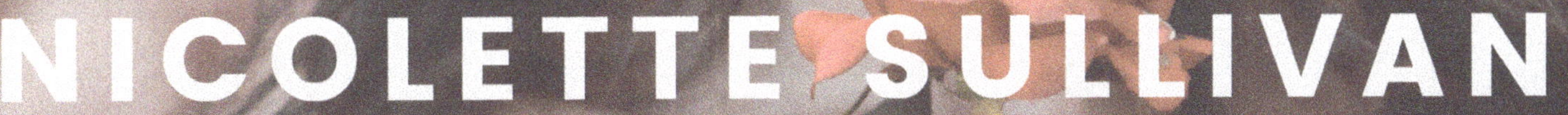

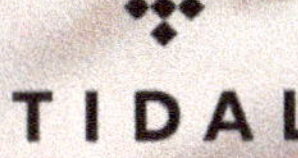

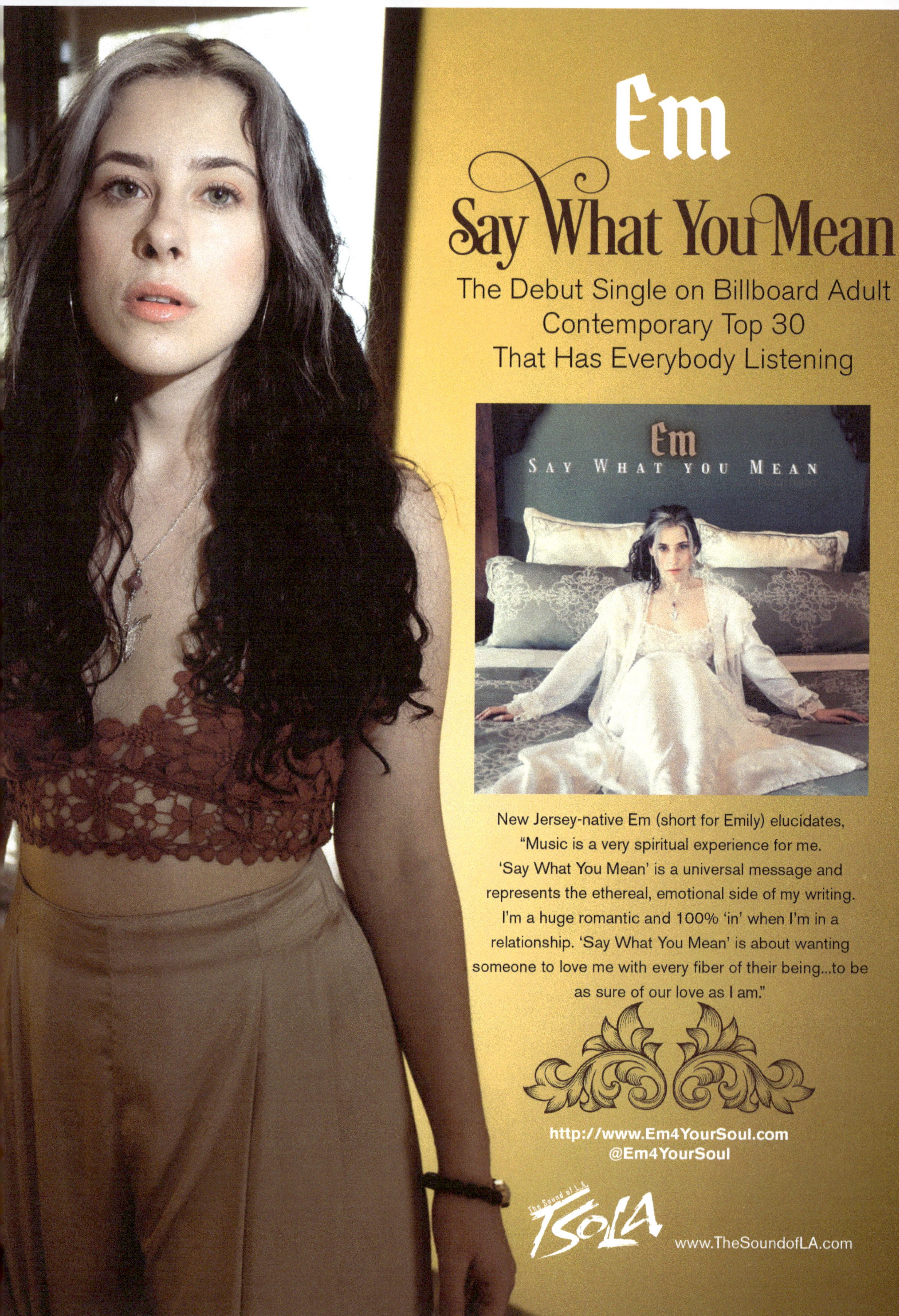
Em

Say What You Mean

The Debut Single on Billboard Adult Contemporary Top 30 That Has Everybody Listening

Em
SAY WHAT YOU MEAN

New Jersey-native Em (short for Emily) elucidates, "Music is a very spiritual experience for me. 'Say What You Mean' is a universal message and represents the ethereal, emotional side of my writing. I'm a huge romantic and 100% 'in' when I'm in a relationship. 'Say What You Mean' is about wanting someone to love me with every fiber of their being...to be as sure of our love as I am."

http://www.Em4YourSoul.com
@Em4YourSoul

The Sound of LA
TSOLA
www.TheSoundofLA.com

WHAT YOU NEED TO KNOW ABOUT THE MUSIC BUSINESS

Whether you are a musician looking to get your band signed or job hunting in the music industry, it's important to understand the full spectrum of the business. When asked how to get in the music industry I tell people to get involved and do "something" yourself that provides value to fans, artists, and music companies. So no matter where you are in your music career this article offers valuable advice for those looking to get in the music industry. Furthermore, you will succeed if you understand the various promotional channels, focus on the right things, and know how to make money in the music business.

WORK HARD

More specifically, work harder than everybody else at the right things. Here is a quote from Caleb Shomo of Beartooth.

"I know so many people that I think could've been some of the biggest acts or some of the best people in this music business and they just didn't really go for it. They kind of waited for it to either fall in their lap or they just let it pass them by and I think it's really important to take opportunities and push for it." – Caleb Shomo of Beartooth – Metal Insider

GET A MENTOR

A mentor doesn't have to be a top industry exec, or even in this industry at all. It doesn't even have to be a face to face relationship. You can get get the same type of advice from books, blogs, video, or interviews with artists or people that you respect. Finally, mentors will keep you honest with yourself, help you stay focused, and contribute to success in business, family life, and health as well.

GETTING MORE FANS

Success starts with your brand and mission. If you don't have your brand and mission, it's too early to start promotional activity.

PUBLICITY

Press, PR, and public relations, are interchangeable terms. Publicists or (PR's) connect your music and brand with all media. Examples: magazines, newspapers, TV, radio interviews (not spinning your track), blogs, podcasts, public appearances (not concerts), sessions, influencers, celebrities, connect with brand partnerships.
The goal of publicity is to spread the artist's vision, accentuate the brand, and draw out the human interest story. They are also responsible for protecting the artist's brand and doing damage control when negative incidents occur. Conversely, they know how to fan the flames when positive events arise. Consequently publicists are experts at "spin", meaning that they can tell your story in different ways depending on the circumstance.

INFLUENCERS

Influencers or social influencers are people who have massive active audiences and with a keyboard or camera can expose their audience to something they like in an instant. Examples of influencers are YouTube vloggers, athletes, celebrities, bloggers, podcasters, or comedians. Most of these influencers have managers, and command high fees. Hiring social influencers is one of the most expensive advertising opportunities I've come across. Influencer costs are 8 to 15 times higher than social media advertising, 5 to 7 times more than banner ad campaigns, and 2 to 4 times higher than magazine print ads. Traffic and impressions sometimes determine the price. But most often it's based on what that particular influencer can command at the moment.

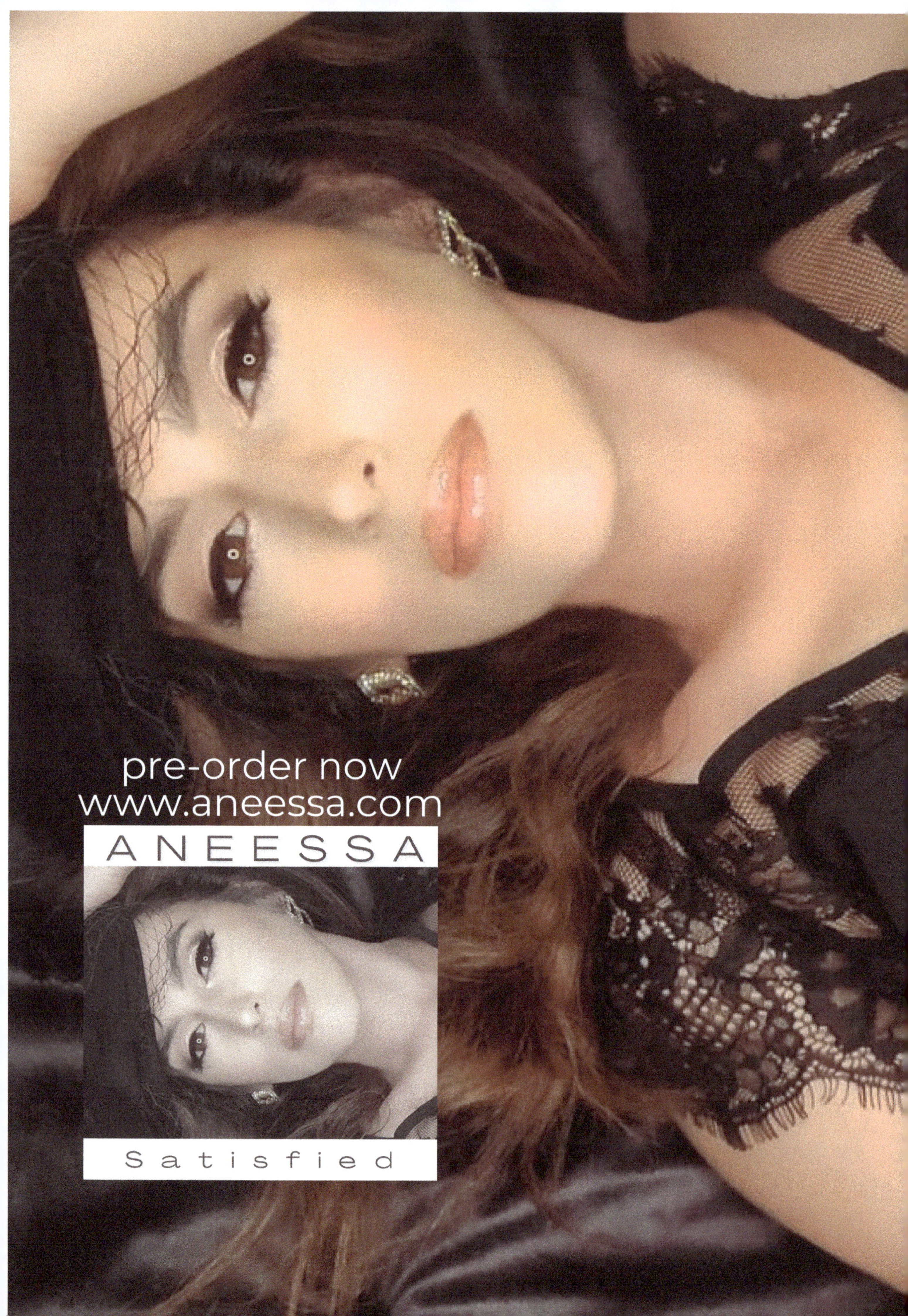

pre-order now
www.aneessa.com
ANEESSA
Satisfied

MINISTER PHYLLIS MCMEANS

"HELP"

A SONG OF HOPE
&
FAITH

PRE-ORDER NOW
IN STORES
FEBRUARY 12

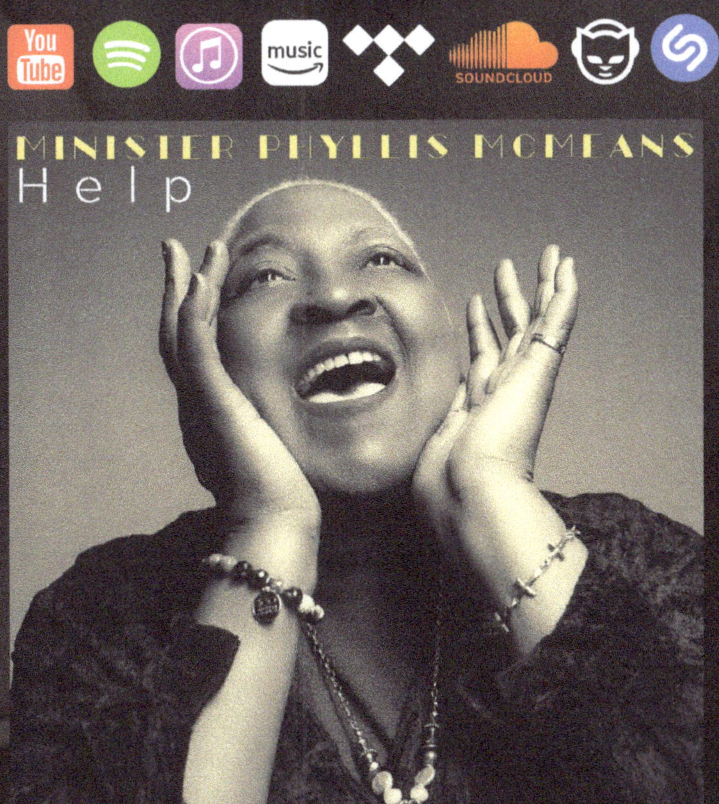

L.A. UNLIMITED

APPAREL REPRESENTATION WITHOUT LIMITS...

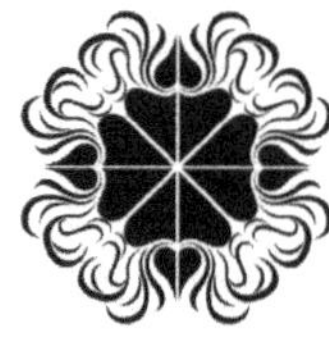

- Corporate Brand Representation
- Brand Identity & Management
- Brand Consulting
- Trade Show Preparation & Participation
- Trunk Shows
- Private Label Sales
- Production Sourcing

L.A. Unlimited & Associates
30765 Pacific Coast Hwy STE
443Malibu, CA 90265

310.882.6432
sales@launlimitedinc.com

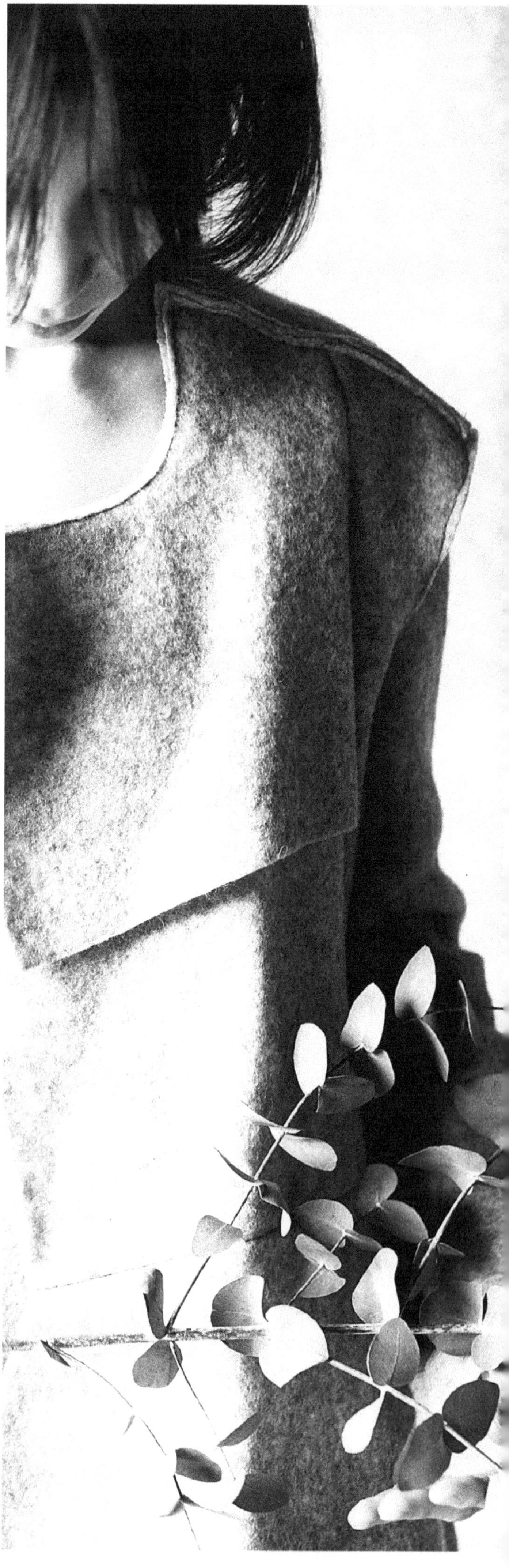

90'S FASHION
IS BACK!

It's no secret: nostalgia sells. And there's no time like the present to feel a little nostalgic.

In fact, we can look forward to emblematic pieces from the '90s trends, such as baggy jeans and the minimalist jewellery given the XXL treatment, coming back into the spotlight.

Don't roll your eyes. 1990s fashion may not be as bad as you and the collective imagination once thought. Yes, the colors were garish. Yes, the cuts were disproportionate. Yes, we have to scour the subject to find the slightest touch of style in the wardrobe of this 'unique' era. But that doesn't prevent us from going back, almost every year, to bring the 90s trends back to life those rare pieces that thrilled a whole generation.

When the present is gloomy and uncertain, we tend to look back at past decades for refuge and set our sights on the one that made us happiest — or is associated with happiness in our memories. Ah, there's nothing like a little nostalgia. And while the '90s trends have long had a bad reputation in terms of fashion, the pieces associated with it remain among the most fun and offbeat in a woman's wardrobe. They are also without a doubt the most comfortable — something that cannot be ignored at the start of this year 2021.

BAGGY IS BACK

Gone are slim- and skinny-cut jeans, which are anyway far too restrictive for our new way of living and working. It's the baggy cut that will be the denim star in 2021. With its ultra-wide legs, it offers absolute comfort without giving up on style — or almost. From Bella Hadid to Hailey Baldwin, many stars have made it their favorite piece of clothing at the beginning of this year, and some fashion addicts have even renamed it "wide-leg jeans" in its most modern version with a higher and less ample waist, to give it a more chic look.

The advantage is that the baggy cut is now available in a wide range of shapes, colors and materials to suit most people. Cargo, perforated, faded, asymmetrical, in leather or imitation leather and even colorful, there is something for all tastes and styles. Worn with sneakers, chunky boots, even heels for the bravest, it will be the centerpiece of your wardrobe until summer.

OVERSIZE JEWELS GO MINIMALIST

Who could forget the big chains worn by rappers in the '90s and 2000s? Well they're making a comeback but in a less blinged-out version. To embellish your most minimalist outfits, homewear or sportswear trends, what could be better than oversized jewellery? In any case, it's what most designers and major brands are betting on at the beginning of this year, in order to put a bit of boldness into your wardrobe.

But be careful not to overdo it. This isn't a reboot of the maximalist trend of recent years. Forget about rhinestones, sequins, and patterns of all kinds, and focus on minimalist models such as bangles, chains, ear studs, or hoops, and adopt them in an XXL format, in gold or silver according to your tastes and desires.

'90S STYLE EVERYWHERE

In fashion, we can also count on seeing the T-shirts, loose shirts and hoodies of the 1990s, but reinterpreted in 2021 style — meaning more feminine, softer, and less… showy. The trend is not new, but rather a natural continuation of the advent of comfortable pieces to wear at home and at work. Unlike in past years, the emphasis will be on the fabric, with a preference for more delicate and refined textiles, or even softer shades, so that chic styles come into play and edge out some of the sportswear inspiration in vogue in recent seasons.

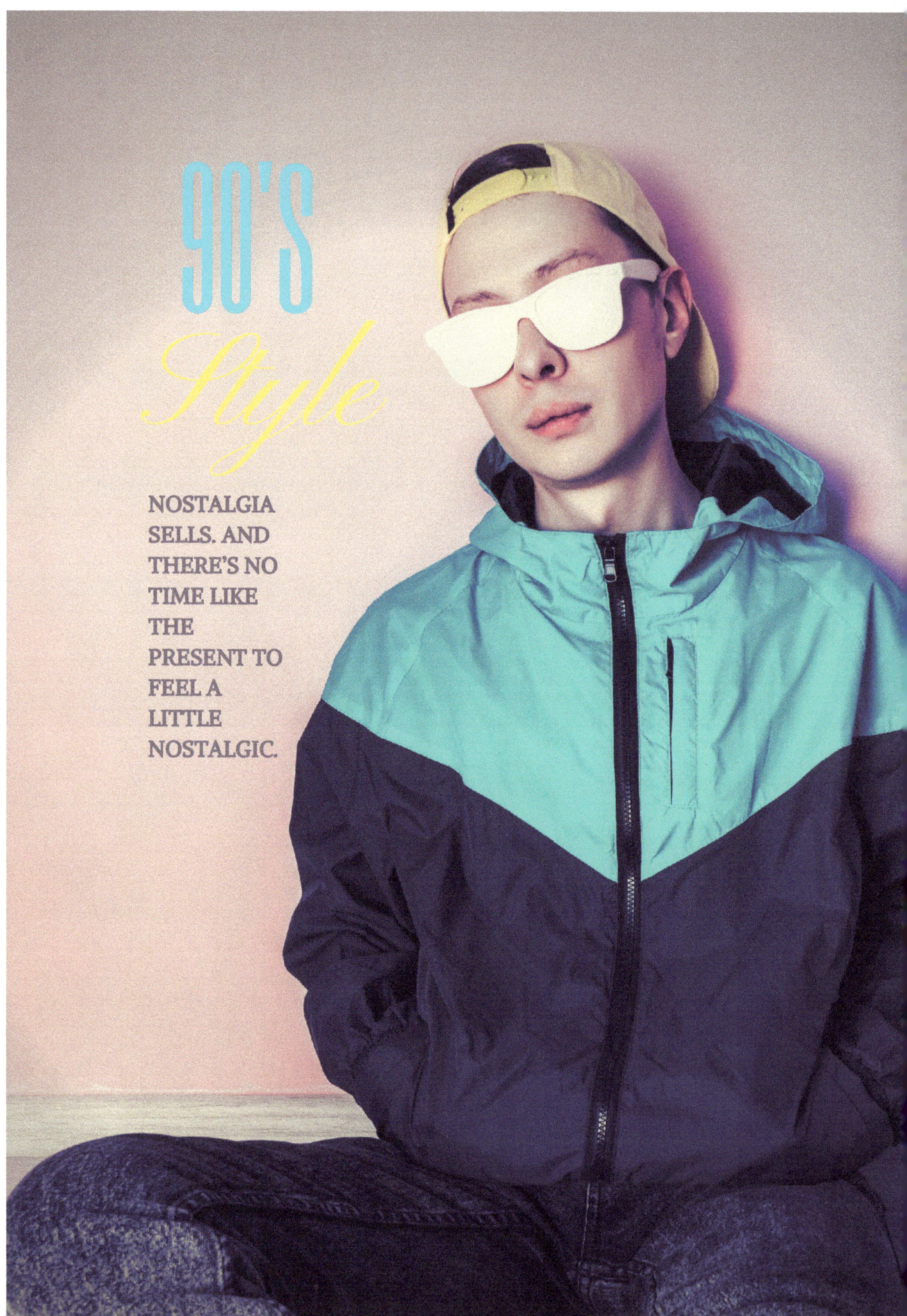

90'S
Style
NOSTALGIA
SELLS. AND
THERE'S NO
TIME LIKE
THE
PRESENT TO
FEEL A
LITTLE
NOSTALGIC.

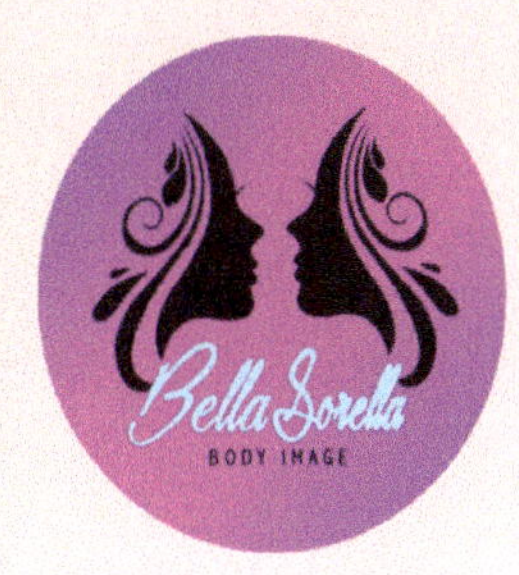

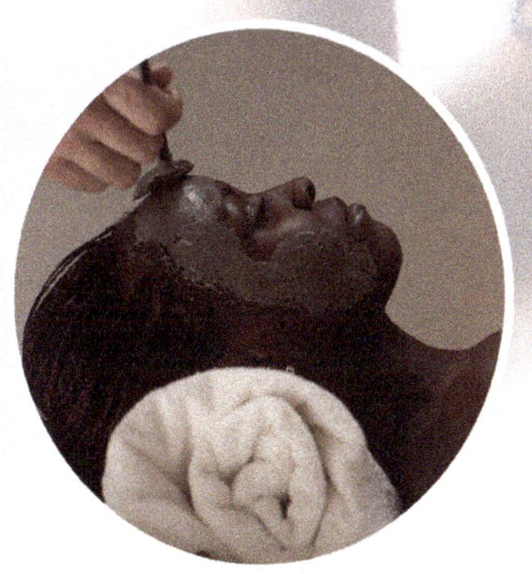

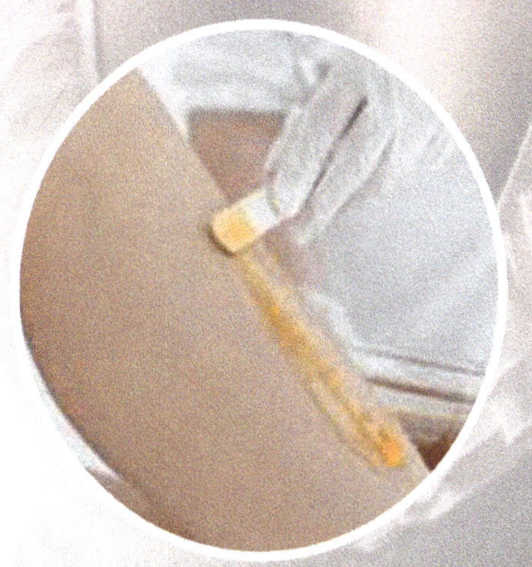

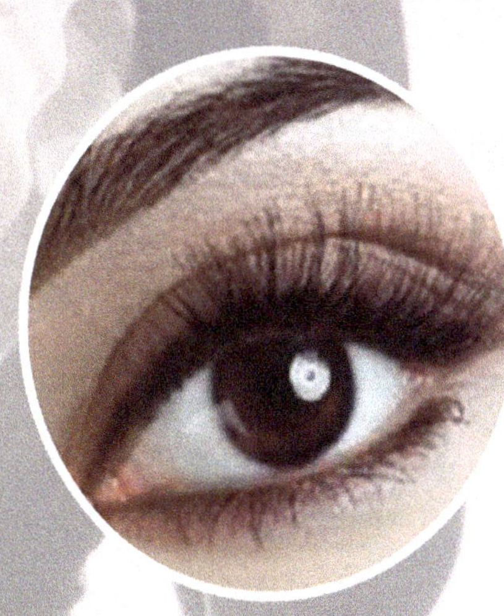

Facial Treatment

Acne - Anti-Ageing - Back
Facial - Hollywood Facial

Waxing

Honey Wax - Stripeless Hard Wax
Gourmet Wax

Lashes & Brows

Lash Tinting
EyeBrow Tinting

More Services

- Microdermabrasion - Dermaplaning
- Chemical Peel - Botox
- Non-invasive Lipo - Non-invasive BBL
- Body Scrub - Body Wrap - Sauna Detox
- Teeth Whitening
  Take-Home Teeth Whitening Kit

Skin & Body Treatment

Enter a world of luxury with the sisters who mastered the world of beauty. Through our carefully crafted services, your mind, body, and soul will obtain results beyond your wildest expectations. We have combined the best artists of beauty in their field with an atmosphere meant to relax and achieve any desired result.

WWW.BELLASORELLABI.COM

2801 South Valley view Blvd. Suite 4, Las Vegas, NV.89102, Tel: 702-530-2615

LED THERAPY

ANTI-AGING TREND

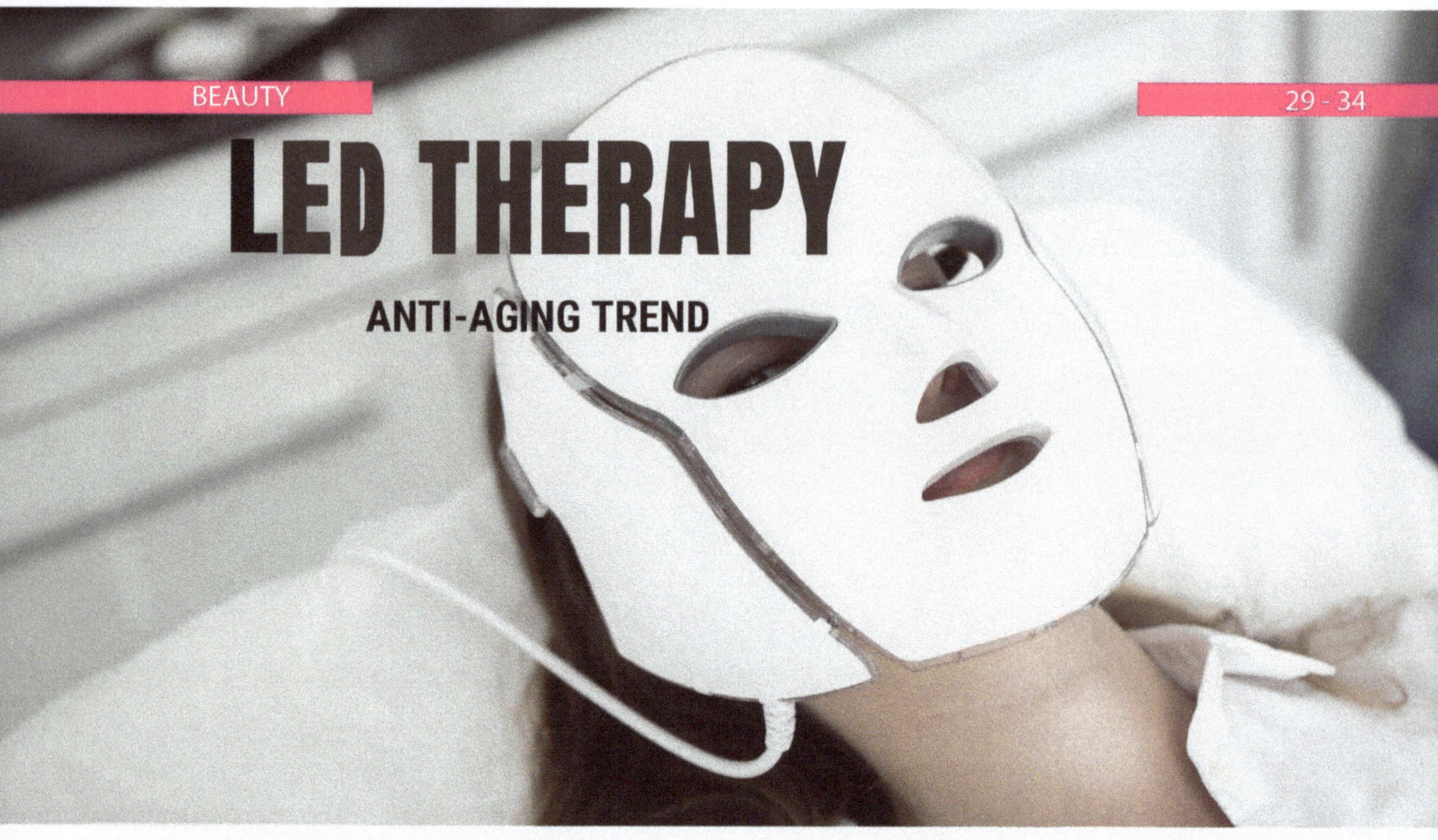

If you've been to a spa, beauty counter, or scrolled through Instagram lately, you've probably seen the unsettling and Michael Myers à la Halloween-esque LED face masks. The devices are kinda creepy, definitely futuristic, and promise all sorts of skin miracles like the reversal of "everything from wrinkles, redness, and signs of aging to acne, scarring, and dark spots," according to Harvard Women's Health Watch. That all sounds great, but the how and why behind all these benefits is far from obvious when looking at the colorful face mask in action. Good thing L'OFFICIEL is here to demystify the process and give so you you all the facts before you consider getting robo-masked up.

LED light therapy, otherwise known as Dermalux™ LED Phototherapy, is a non-invasive skin rejuvenation treatment. Using a narrow band of non-thermal LED light energy, the procedure stimulates your body's natural cell production for an accelerated repair of the skin's surface. By speeding up skin's regenerative process, evidence of sun damage, acne, inflammation, or even more serious conditions like eczema, psoriasis, dermatitis, and rosacea is reduced. For people with wounds or other kinds of scarring, the regrowth of skin cells as promoted by LED Phototherapy can also be curative.
Though, it's important to note that these healing results take time and consistent regimens of treatments. A single LED facial will reduce inflammation, skin irritation, and boost the natural glow of skin, sure. But to see scars disappear, treat acne, or reduce wrinkles, the American Academy of Dermatology recommends at least several weeks of consistent sessions to start seeing results. Consistency ensures the progressive penetration of the LED light deeper and deeper into the skin with each new treatment. When new depths are reached by the light, more corrective results can be achieved.

Understanding your specific skin goals is also crucial to tailoring the LED light experience to your individual needs. There are three kinds of LED light: blue light, red light, and near infa-red light, each designed for different results. Blue light is an antibacterial treatment intended to address acne by reducing oil production and preventing future breakouts, without irritating skin. This colorwave is also a UV-free alternative to treating eczema and psoriasis. Red light increases skin's hydration, reduces inflammation, redness, and the appearance of pores. Similar to blue light, red light can regulate skin oil, as well as increase the circulation of other vital fluids in order to speed up the repair of skin and correct rosacea (as medically-approved by your dermatologist, of course). Near infa-red light is the most intense form of LED Phototherapy, and reaches farther into the skin than the other two colorwaves. This color treatment is meant to increase the absorption capabilities of cells, smooth signs of age, and improve the elasticity of skin. It is also used to accelerate the healing process of cystic acne or wounds.

HOW TO RAPIDLY GROW
YOUR INSTAGRAM FOLLOWING

Do you need to "know somebody" or "get lucky" to build a fan base and grow an income as an artist?
Absolutely not!

RESEARCH AND INCORPORATE RELEVANT HASHTAGS

Now that you're tracking your retargetable engagement, the next step is to find relevant hashtags for your business.
Open Instagram and navigate to the Search & Explore tab. Start by searching for one hashtag such as #independentartist
You likely have a core group of hashtags you're already using in your own posts. Because it's best to search and engage daily, I recommend that you set up a spreadsheet to track all of the relevant hashtags you're using because the list will quickly grow.

IDENTIFY AND ENGAGE WITH 9 RELEVANT INSTAGRAM POSTS

Take a few seconds to analyze each Instagram post you come across. I recommend clicking the full post to:
Read the caption.
Quickly measure the engagement rate (likes and comments vs. total followers).
Click the account profile image to check out their bio and the rest of their profile.
Remember, this strategy works across any vertical: B2B, B2C, SMB, etc. It's the process of culling through the noise to find the gems that most of your competitors aren't setting aside enough time to do.

 Share your own experiences. Is there something in your life (or behind the scenes in your business) that's relatable to the original caption? Share that!

Ask open-ended questions. The goal here is to get people to come back to your Instagram profile and engage. If you only talk about yourself and your own experiences, it lessens your chance of developing a meaningful conversation with the other person.

Don't be a know-it-all. Let other people share their perspective and worldview. We, as humans, love to share about ourselves often. Remember that this exercise is not about YOU. It's about the incredible humans you serve in your marketing.

MONETIZE YOUR EFFORTS WITH AN AD SEQUENCE

After going through these steps, you've started to build two powerful marketing assets:

A captive community of current and future customers who drive real revenue
An engaged custom audience available for retargeting with paid advertising
The first of these two assets, a captive community, will fuel your organic Instagram efforts again and again. Next time you publish a post, these followers will be hungry for your new content. Because you've now engaged in conversations with these users, they're more ready to engage and respond than total strangers.

The second asset is an engaged custom audience that's retargetable by building a $5/day Instagram ad campaign.

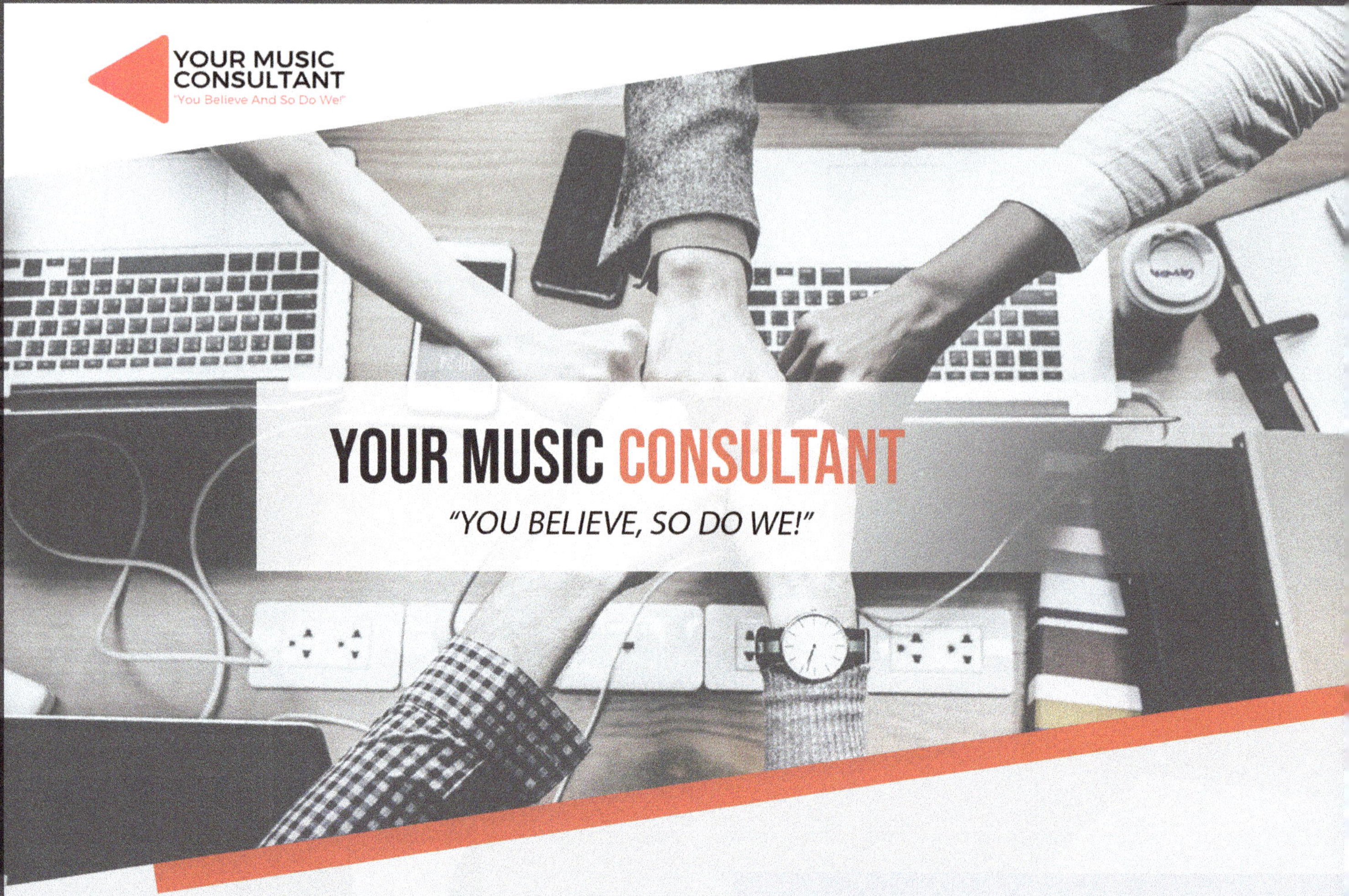

YOUR MUSIC CONSULTANT

"YOU BELIEVE, SO DO WE!"

We Can Help You To Grow Your Business

We are a monthly based service, we put faith in artists who has major potential, believed in them, and who are willing to spend their time and own money to work with us in building a successful music career!

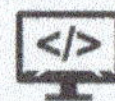

Digital Marketing Services

SOCIAL MEDIA - STREAMING SERVICES - MUSIC DISTRIBUTION - PRESS RELEASE - PRESS DISTRIBUTION - PR

Radio Airplay and TV Commercial

TERRESTRIAL AND DIGITAL RADIO CAMPAIGN AL GENRES EXCEPT HEAVY METAL - CABLE TV AND MAJOR NETWORK COMMERCIAL

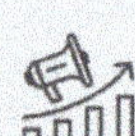

Licensing & Booking

CONCERTS, LIVE MUSIC, EVENTS, CLUB NIGHTS - RED CARPETS - FOREIGN LICENSING AND SUB0PUBLISHING

Why Choose Us ?

3 DECADES OF MUSIC BUSINESS EXPERIENCE
Platinium and Gold Records
MOTOWN RECORDS
UNIVERSAL
SONY
CAPITOL RECORDS

WE WORKED WITH:
Kanye West - Jay Z - Stevie Wonder - Michael Jackson - Germaine Jackson Smokey Robinson - Dionne Warwick - Cheryl Lynn - The Originals -

📞 **1 -818-514-0038**
(Ext. 1)
Monday - Friday / 9am to 6pm

FIND US :

www.YourMusicConsultant.com
30721 Russell Ranch Road Suite 140 Westlake Village, USA
Email : info@yourmusicconsultant.com

MUSIC DOCUMENTARIES
2021

The music documentary resurgence is alive and well and set to continue into 2021 with an insatiable appetite for weird and wild movies about bands and artists.

TINA TURNER

The Private Dancer star is getting the feature treatment from the filmmakers behind Searching For Sugar Man, Whitney and LA92. Directed by TJ Martin and Dan Lindsay and produced by Simon and Jonathan Chinn's Lightbox, the film is set to air on HBO in the U.S. and Sky in the UK. It will tell of Turner's career, from starting out in The Ike & Tina Turner Revue through to becoming one of the biggest-selling solo performers in the world, via a tumultuous marriage. The film will feature interviews with Turner and her friends and collaborators and is set to include previously unseen footage.

SUMMER OF SOUL (…OR, WHEN THE REVOLUTION COULD NOT BE TELEVISED)

Premiering at Sundance 2021 is Questlove's directorial debut, Summer of Soul (…Or, When The Revolution Could Not Be Televised). The film features unearthed footage from the Harlem Cultural Festival that has sat in a basement unseen for 50 years. The festival was attended by over 300,000, taking place the same summer as Woodstock, celebrating African American music and culture, and promoting Black pride and unity. The film, which previously had a working title of Black Woodstock, is produced by David Dinerstein, Robert Fyvolent and Joseph Patel. The Roots drummer/frontman Questlove, otherwise known as Ahmir Thompson, said he was "damn proud" of it.

THE SPARKS BROTHERS

Edgar Wright is best known for directing films such as Baby Driver and Shaun of the Dead. But he is now making his documentary directorial debut with a film about "This Town Ain't Big Enough For The Both Of Us" rockers Sparks. The film, which is also set to premiere at Sundance, will look at how the quirky band, featuring brothers Ron & Russell Mael, is successful, underrated, hugely influential, and criminally overlooked all at the same time. The film, which has been in the works for the past few years, includes vintage film footage of the band as well as footage of their show at the Kentish Town Forum in 2018. Wright said the film would be a "musical odyssey through five weird and wonderful decades" on "your favorite band's favorite band."y.

BILLIE EILISH: THE WORLD'S A LITTLE BLURRY

Press, PR, and public relations, are interchangeable terms. Publicists or (PR's) connect your music and Music documentaries have become big business – particularly if they feature an A-list artist at the top of their game. Apple TV+ paid around $26 million for the Billie Eilish: The World's a Little Blurry, a film about the "Bad Guy" singer. The film will tell the story of the teenage phenomenon, who has broken through to become one of the hottest pop stars in the world thanks to her songs and a don't-give-a-f*ck attitude. Directed by Belushi and The September Issue director R.J. Cutler, the film will premiere in February and is produced by Cutler's This Machine in association with Interscope Films, Eilish label Darkroom and Lighthouse Management & Media, run by manager Aleen Keshishian.

LITTLE RICHARD

Jerry Lee Lewis' good friend Little Richard, who died earlier this year, is also getting the doc treatment with a new film from All In: The Fight for Democracy director Lisa Cortes and executive producer Dee Rees (Mudbound). The film will tell the story of the man known as the Innovator, the Originator and the Architect of rock n roll.

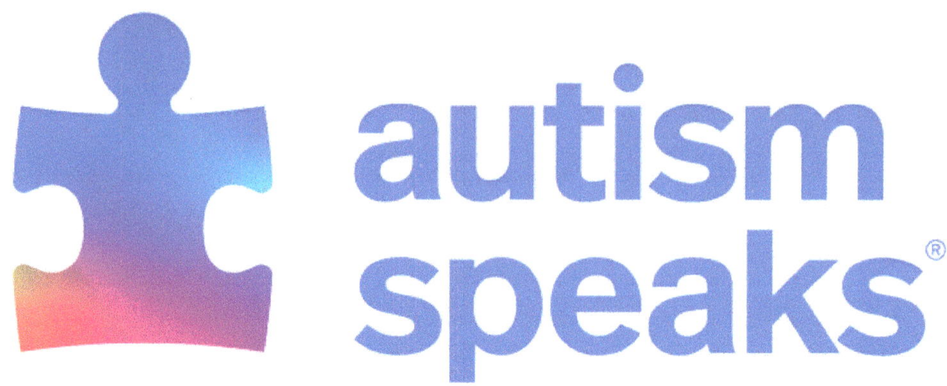

Autism Speaks Walk is the world's largest autism fundraising event dedicated to improving the lives of people with autism. Powered by the love of people with autism and the parents, grandparents, siblings, friends, relatives and providers who support them, the funds raised help ensure people of all abilities have access to the tools needed to lead 'their best lives.'

The commitment of individuals like you plays a critical role in raising the funding needed to fuel innovative research and lifelong supports and services. Working together, there is no limit to what we can achieve. Please register and fundraise for an Autism Speaks Walk near you.

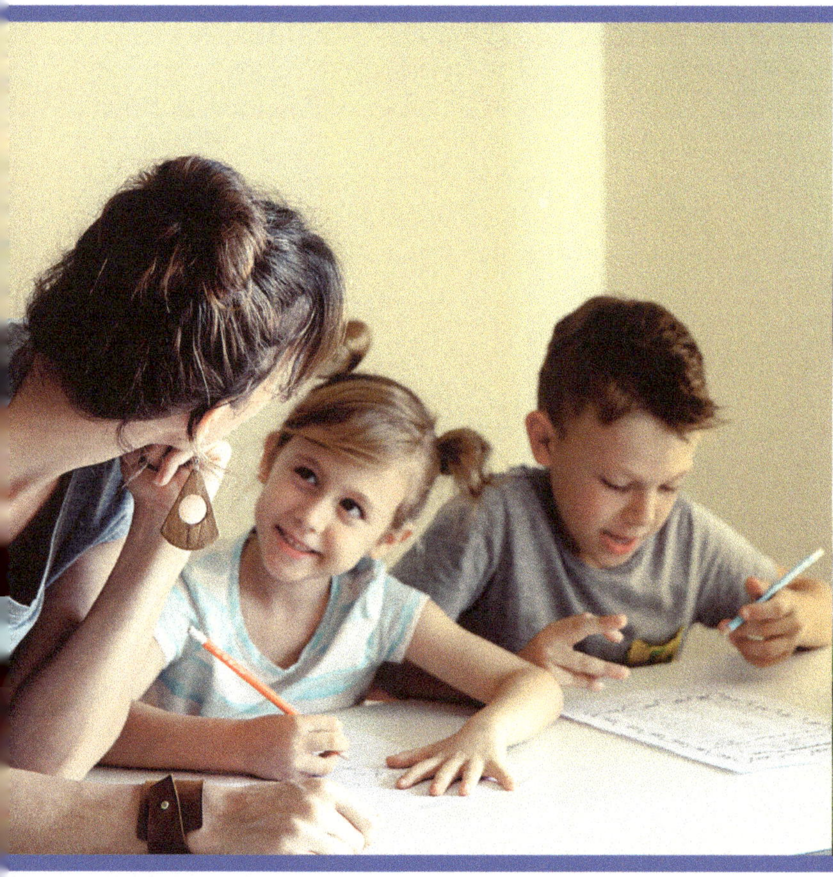

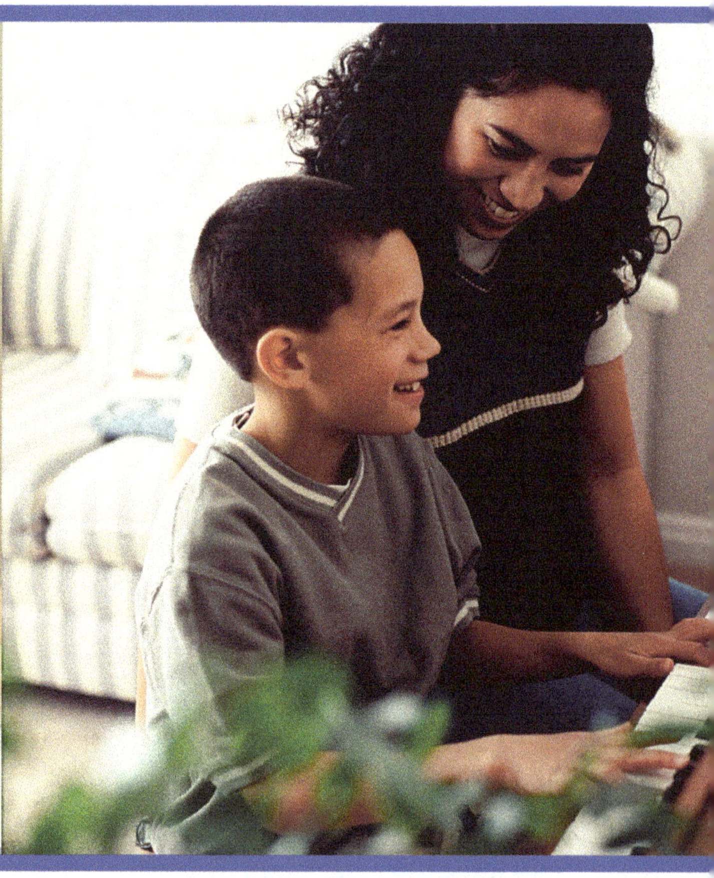

To learn more about autism, visit www.AutismSpeaks.org or contact our Autism Response Team at 888-288-4762 or en Español 888-772-9050,

www.ingramcontent.com/pod-product-compliance
Lightning Source LLC
Chambersburg PA
CBHW041352050726
47599CB00016B/1861